The Caregiver

In the

Rehabilitation

Department

MARTIN STERLING

Table of contents

Introduction: The core business of the rehabilitation department — 15

- The importance of the caregiver's role in the rehabilitation process. — 16
- The changing role of the nursing auxiliary in the face of rehabilitation — 18
- Presentation of the general framework of the book. — 20

Chapter 1: Understanding the rehabilitation department: A unique environment — 23

Definition and role of rehabilitation in the healthcare system — 24

- Rehabilitation: between acute care and return to autonomy. — 24
- The department's specific features compared with other units. — 26

The different types of rehabilitation — 28

- Functional rehabilitation: neurological, orthopedic, cardiac, respiratory. — 28

- ○ Post-trauma and post-surgical rehabilitation. 31

Multidisciplinary teamwork 33

- ○ The caregiver's place in the medical team: doctors, physiotherapists, occupational therapists. 33
- ○ Interactions with patients and families. 36

The specific missions of the rehabilitation orderly 38

- ○ Ensure the well-being and clinical monitoring of patients. 38
- ○ Facilitate patients' rehabilitation and reintegration into everyday life. 41

Chapter 2: Welcoming and assessing the patient : The crucial observation stage 45

Reception in the rehabilitation department: A key moment 46

- ○ Care on arrival: listening and humanity. 46
- ○ Creating a safe, reassuring environment. 48

Day-to-day clinical observation 50

- Recognize signs of improvement or complications. — 50
- Tools for monitoring and communicating with the care team. — 53

The caregiver's role in assessing patient autonomy — 56

- Autonomy evaluation grids and their use. — 56
- Participate in adjusting the care plan according to the patient's progress. — 59

Chapter 3: Supporting basic care in a rehabilitation context — 63

Hygiene care for rehabilitation patients — 64

- Body hygiene: adapting care to physical limitations. — 64
- Prevention of pressure sores and other complications associated with immobility. — 66

Assistance with mobilization and pain management — 69

- Techniques to assist mobilization without aggravating lesions. — 69

- Pain monitoring and collaboration with the team for relief. ... 72

Nutrition and hydration for rehabilitation patients ... 75

- Adapt meals to the patient's condition: assistance, monitoring of specific diets. ... 75
- Promote independent eating while maintaining safety. ... 78

Chapter 4: Taking an active part in the rehabilitation process ... 81

Collaboration with physiotherapists and occupational therapists ... 82

- Help in preparing rehabilitation sessions. ... 82
- Effort monitoring and support for rehabilitation activities. ... 84

Encouraging and motivating patients on a daily basis ... 87

- Strategies to boost patient motivation. ... 87
- Dealing with frustrations and psychological blockages. ... 90

Psychosocial rehabilitation ... 93

- The caregiver's role in psychological support. ... 93

- Help rebuild self-esteem and independence. — 96

Chapter 5: Specific pathologies and their impact on rehabilitation — 99

Stroke and neurological rehabilitation — 100

- The role of the caregiver in motor and cognitive recovery. — 100
- Challenges specific to patients suffering from aphasia or — 102

Post-operative rehabilitation: Orthopedic and cardio-respiratory surgery — 105

- Supporting patients who have undergone prostheses, complex fractures or coronary bypass surgery. — 105
- Specific monitoring and management of post-operative complications. — 108

Patients suffering from chronic illnesses: diabetes, kidney failure, etc. — 111

- How to adapt care and exercise to chronic pathologies. — 111
- The link between rehabilitation and the prevention of chronic disease complications. — 114

Chapter 6: Managing young and pediatric rehabilitation patients   119

Special care for children   120

- Adapting care and communication to the needs of children in rehabilitation.   120
- The role of the caregiver in supporting psychomotor development.   123

Supporting young adults and teenagers   125

- Take into account the identity and emotional issues of young patients.   125
- Helping young people recovering from illness to return to school or work.   128

Support for parents and relatives of paediatric patients   131

- Manage parents' anxiety and involve them in care without overburdening them.   131
- The importance of creating an environment of trust for the child and his family.   134

Chapter 7: New technologies for rehabilitation — 137

Telerehabilitation: a fast-growing alternative — 138

- How telerehabilitation can support remote patient monitoring. — 138
- The role of the caregiver in using communication technologies to maintain a link with the patient. — 140

Digital mobility assessment tools — 143

- Use connected applications and tools to assess patient progress (activity bracelets, movement sensors). — 143
- Monitor health indicators using computerized, interconnected patient records. — 146

Artificial intelligence and rehabilitation: what place for the caregiver? — 149

- The impact of new technologies on care and rehabilitation methods. — 149
- The importance of keeping up to date with technological advances to optimize patient care. — 153

Conclusion: A vocation in the service of rehabilitation   157

- Summary of challenges and rewards.   158

- Encouragement and a call to commit to this rewarding path.   160

Appendices : Practical resources and tools   163

- Practical data sheets: protocols, mobilization techniques, evaluation grids.   163

« The rehabilitation department is not simply a place for physical care, but a space where dignity, autonomy and hope are rebuilt. The caregiver's every gesture becomes an essential link in the process of the patient's reappropriation of body and mind. »

Introduction

The core business in the rehabilitation department

- The importance of the caregiver's role in the rehabilitation process.

The importance of the caregiver's role in the rehabilitation process cannot be underestimated, as he or she is a central pillar of the recovery process. The caregiver is at the heart of the patient's day-to-day physical and psychological care. In the rehabilitation department, the patient is no longer simply being treated for an acute pathology, but is engaged in a long and complex process aimed at restoring his or her autonomy and quality of life. This is where the caregiver comes in, with a role that goes far beyond basic care.

From the moment the patient is admitted, the caregiver plays a vital role in establishing a climate of trust. Patients, often weakened by illness or surgery, must not only accept the physical limitations imposed by their state of health, but also commit to a demanding rehabilitation program. The caregiver's direct, regular contact with the patient provides a stable, reassuring point of reference. They provide a permanent link between the patient and the nursing team, closely observing the slightest changes in the patient's physical and emotional state.

In the context of rehabilitation, hygiene and comfort care, one of the caregiver's key skills, take on a special dimension. The aim is not only to ensure the patient's immediate well-being, but also to help him or her progress towards greater autonomy. On a daily basis, the caregiver must assess the patient's ability to perform everyday tasks, such as dressing, washing or moving around, and adapt his or her assistance accordingly. For example, at the start of the program, the patient may need total assistance to wash, but the aim is to enable him or her, over time, to regain a degree of independence, even if only partial. This evolution is at the heart of the caregiver's work, who encourages and motivates the patient every step of the way, while respecting his or her limits.

The caregiver's psychological support is also essential. Rehabilitation can be a long and frustrating process. Some patients have to relearn basic functions, such as walking or talking, which can generate a profound sense of discouragement. The caregiver's constant presence becomes a source of comfort. They know how to listen, soothe and encourage the patient to persevere, even in difficult times. This close relationship enables the caregiver to understand the patient's fears and emotional needs, thus fostering a more holistic and humane approach to care.

On a technical level, the nursing auxiliary works closely with the rehabilitation team, in particular physiotherapists and occupational therapists. They take an active part in rehabilitation sessions, helping to prepare the patient, mobilizing him or her or observing the efforts made. His role is also to watch for signs of fatigue or pain that could limit the patient's progress. They are often the first to alert the medical team to subtle changes in the patient's condition, as their daily observation enables them to pick up on details that may escape the notice of other team members.

The caregiver is also the person who ensures the patient's safety throughout his or her stay. Rehabilitation patients are often vulnerable to falls or complications arising from prolonged immobility. Through regular interventions, the caregiver implements appropriate preventive measures, whether it's repositioning a bedridden patient to prevent bedsores, or accompanying a patient as he or she takes his or her first steps after surgery. These seemingly simple gestures have a major impact on care quality and patient safety.

Finally, the caregiver contributes to the patient's gradual autonomy by helping them to regain confidence in their abilities. Each small step forward, each more autonomous gesture, is a shared victory between patient and caregiver. The caregiver's constant encouragement plays a key role in motivating the patient to persevere. It's not just a question of technical care, but of a human accompaniment that gives the patient the tools to reclaim his or her body and regain an active place in society.

- The changing role of the nursing auxiliary in the face of rehabilitation challenges.

The evolution of the nursing profession in the face of rehabilitation challenges reflects the profound changes taking place in the healthcare system, and the growing expectations placed on care professionals. Historically focused on hygiene and comfort tasks, the caregiver's role has expanded over the decades to become a key player in the rehabilitation process, an increasingly strategic field as the population ages and rehabilitation needs grow.

In the context of rehabilitation, the nursing profession has taken on a new dimension. Previously seen primarily as a support to nurses in providing basic care, the nursing auxiliary now plays an active and indispensable role in helping patients to become autonomous. Medical advances are saving more and more lives, but these medical victories often require long and complex rehabilitation to enable the patient to regain an acceptable quality of life. Caregivers must therefore adapt to these new realities and develop specific skills to meet the demands of this rehabilitation.

One of the main aspects of this evolution is the diversification of the rehabilitation caregiver's missions. Whereas they traditionally provided assistance with hygiene, comfort and nutrition, caregivers are now involved in more technical and complex tasks. They play an active role in the clinical monitoring of patients, identifying signs of improvement or, on the contrary, complications likely to slow down rehabilitation. Through careful observation, the nursing auxiliary becomes a genuine relay between the patient and the multidisciplinary team, transmitting essential information that enables care and rehabilitation plans to be adjusted.

This role as intermediary between patient and care team underlines another major development: the rehabilitation caregiver must not only master basic care, but also develop an in-depth understanding of specific pathologies, rehabilitation processes, as well as mobilization and functional rehabilitation techniques. The diversity of rehabilitation patients, whether they have suffered a stroke, undergone major surgery or are recovering from a long illness, requires the caregiver to have a finer level of expertise. This requires ongoing training and the ability to constantly adapt to evolving care techniques.

At the same time, the caregiver is faced with ever-increasing psychosocial challenges. Rehabilitation is not just a physical process, but also a mental one. Many patients, particularly those who have suffered a significant loss of function, find themselves in a state of psychological vulnerability, faced with the uncertainty of their future or the anxiety of not being able to regain their autonomy. In this context, the caregiver is no longer content with ensuring immediate well-being, but must also play a moral support role, encouraging patients to overcome their fears and persevere despite the obstacles. This relational and psychological dimension of the job has intensified, requiring more developed communication and empathy skills.

Another important development is the growing use of technology in rehabilitation. Caregivers must adapt to the integration of digital tools, remote monitoring devices and high-tech rehabilitation equipment, such as exoskeletons and virtual reality systems used for motor rehabilitation. This technological revolution, while providing innovative solutions to accelerate patient recovery, requires caregivers to master tools that were not necessary in the past. Caregivers are called upon to train themselves in the use of these new technologies, in order to provide patients with the best possible support in their care, and to optimize the rehabilitation process.

Finally, the evolution of the nursing profession is also taking place in a context where public health policies are emphasizing the importance of rehabilitation to reduce the length of hospital stays and encourage patients to return home. This means that caregivers must not only accompany patients within the hospital or rehabilitation facilities, but also prepare them for discharge, by teaching them essential gestures to live independently or semi-autonomously. The caregiver must therefore work closely with social workers, families and the patients themselves to ensure that the necessary conditions for a successful discharge are in place, while anticipating any rehabilitation needs at home.

This evolution is accompanied by increasing reflection on the value of the caregiver's skills and his or her role in the multidisciplinary team. The profession is no longer limited to supportive care: it is part of a broader therapeutic dynamic, in which the caregiver becomes a fully-fledged player in the patient's functional recovery and reintegration into daily life. This recognition must be achieved through better initial training, as well as through specialization courses in rehabilitation, to equip caregivers with the tools and know-how they need to meet current and future challenges in this field.

- Presentation of the general framework of the book.

This book is an in-depth, practical exploration of the caregiver's role in rehabilitation, a field where patient care is not limited to comfort care, but is part of an overall process of recovery, rehabilitation and reintegration. Aimed directly at students, novice caregivers and those wishing to deepen their skills in this specific field, this book aims to offer a comprehensive and realistic vision of daily life in rehabilitation, while providing concrete tools to excel in this environment.

The general framework of this book is based on the idea that the rehabilitation department is a unique environment, where every gesture, every intervention, is crucial to the patient's progress. Here, the nursing auxiliary is not simply a care provider, but a key player in the therapeutic process. Although often regarded as an auxiliary role, this profession is actually at the heart of the recovery process for patients following physical trauma, major surgery or chronic illness.

The book's approach is resolutely practical, but rooted in the reality of the field. Far from offering abstract theory, it delves into the day-to-day challenges of the rehabilitation department. Readers will discover the specific tasks, the essential technical and relational skills, and the ethical dilemmas facing caregivers in this type of service. The book also highlights the importance of constant adaptation to evolving patient needs and medical and technological advances, as rehabilitation is a field in constant transformation.

The aim is to prepare the reader for the complex and demanding reality of this environment, by providing both essential theoretical knowledge and concrete examples drawn from the day-to-day experience of professionals. In a clear progression, the book begins with the fundamentals of the rehabilitation service, then goes on to detail the different types of care, specific pathologies and the essential role of the nursing auxiliary within a multidisciplinary team. Each chapter deals with a specific aspect of the profession, from patient reception and hygiene management to active participation in rehabilitation, psychological support and ethical and technical issues.

This book does more than simply provide a description of the tasks involved; it invites the reader to reflect on the evolution of the profession, the impact of new technologies on rehabilitation, and the growing role of the caregiver in a healthcare system where patient autonomy is a central objective. In this sense, it highlights the role of the caregiver as facilitator of autonomy, in collaboration with physiotherapists, occupational therapists and the entire medical team.

Particular attention is also paid to the human side of the profession. The book underlines the extent to which interpersonal skills, emotional management and empathy are essential to successful rehabilitation work. Patients undergoing rehabilitation are often faced with physical and mental limitations that profoundly affect their daily lives. The caregiver, in constant interaction with the patient, becomes a crucial psychological support, in addition to ensuring quality care. The book places great emphasis on the helping relationship and the caregiver's role in managing patients' moments of doubt, frustration or discouragement.

In short, this book is destined to become an essential reference for those wishing to move into the rehabilitation service, or for professionals already in the field who are looking to deepen their knowledge. It offers a rich and nuanced vision of this rapidly evolving profession, where care is not limited to technique, but encompasses a genuine approach to patient support and reintegration. Whether it's helping patients regain their autonomy after an accident, operation or chronic illness, or supporting their morale in the face of the trials of rehabilitation, the caregiver is at the center of this complex and essential care pathway.

Chapter 1

Understanding the rehabilitation department: A unique environment

Definition and role of rehabilitation in the healthcare system

- Rehabilitation: between acute care and return to autonomy.

Rehabilitation occupies a unique place in the care process, at the crossroads between acute care and the return to autonomy. It is a pivotal stage that takes place after the critical phase of an illness, operation or trauma, when the vital emergency has been brought under control, but the patient remains vulnerable and often limited in his or her functional abilities. The rehabilitation department is distinguished by its fundamental aim: to help patients restore their physical, cognitive and social independence. Here, the main challenge is to enable each individual to regain maximum autonomy, adapted to his or her abilities and life goals, whether this involves resuming a professional activity, returning to the home, or simply reacquainting oneself with the essential gestures of daily life.

Rehabilitation often begins after a period of hospitalization in acute care, where the focus is on medical stabilization and immediate treatment of the pathology. Here, care teams intervene primarily to meet the patient's urgent needs, whether to treat an infection, perform surgery or stabilize a vital function. Once this critical phase is over, the patient, although medically cured, often remains weakened and limited in his or her ability to function independently. This is when rehabilitation takes over.

This transition from acute care to rehabilitation is a key step. While intensive or acute care focuses on survival, rehabilitation aims to give patients back the means to live life to the full, according to their new capacities. It is based on a holistic, multidisciplinary approach, mobilizing several healthcare professionals such as rehabilitation physicians, physiotherapists, occupational therapists, speech therapists, psychologists and, of course, care assistants. Together, they work with the patient to draw up an individualized rehabilitation plan, tailored to his or her specific needs and functional objectives.

At the heart of this process, rehabilitation focuses on re-training the patient in essential gestures that may seem trivial, but which are the basis of autonomy. For some, this may mean relearning to walk after surgery or an accident; for others, it may mean regaining the ability to feed oneself, wash or dress oneself. The rehabilitation process varies according to pathologies and after-effects, but the principle remains the same: each stage aims to reduce the patient's dependence on carers, by progressively reinforcing his or her physical and mental capacities.

The importance of rehabilitation also lies in its individualized approach. Unlike acute care, where medical intervention is often standardized to respond rapidly to emergency situations, rehabilitation takes into account the specific features of each patient. The care team assesses not only physical limitations, but also the cognitive, emotional and social aspects that can influence the recovery process. Some patients may be reluctant to undergo rehabilitation, either because they underestimate their abilities, or because they are discouraged by the slow pace of progress. This is where human support, particularly that provided by caregivers, plays a crucial role. Through their daily proximity to the patient, caregivers provide a reassuring presence, motivating and encouraging every little bit of progress.

Rehabilitation is not just about physical rehabilitation. It also encompasses mental and emotional rehabilitation, as the rehabilitation journey is often fraught with psychological obstacles. Patients faced with new, even temporary, disabilities may suffer from mood disorders, depression or anxiety linked to the uncertainty of their recovery. The aim of rehabilitation is therefore also to restore self-confidence and hope, and to help patients regain their psychological equilibrium.

In addition, the success of rehabilitation depends to a large extent on continuity of care and preparation for the return home. For some patients, the rehabilitation process may continue long after they have left the rehabilitation center, requiring follow-up care at home or on an outpatient basis. Care assistants, in collaboration with other team members, play a central role in this preparation. They help to educate the patient and his or her family, teaching them the techniques and precautions to follow to ensure the patient's safety and autonomy at home.

The return to autonomy is not always total, especially in cases where the after-effects of a pathology are permanent. However, rehabilitation aims to maximize the patient's independence within the limits of his or her abilities, by offering the necessary tools to adapt his or her lifestyle to his or her new reality. In some cases, this may involve the use of technical aids, such as walkers or prostheses, or adaptations to the home environment, to facilitate movement or everyday gestures. The ultimate aim is to enable the patient to regain a certain quality of life, and reduce his or her dependence on caregivers as much as possible.

- The department's specific features compared with other units.

The rehabilitation department differs fundamentally from other medical units in its holistic approach and the very nature of the care it provides. Unlike acute care services, such as emergency or surgery, where the aim is to quickly stabilize the patient's state of health and treat an immediate pathology, the rehabilitation service takes a longer view, with a central objective: to restore the patient's ability to reappropriate his or her body and its essential functions, in order to restore autonomy as far as possible.

One of the key features of this department is its multidisciplinary nature. In contrast to conventional medical units, where intervention is mainly centered around one specialty (e.g. cardiology or neurology), the rehabilitation department relies on close, ongoing collaboration between different healthcare professionals. Alongside rehabilitation doctors and nurses, there are physiotherapists, occupational therapists, speech therapists, psychologists, social workers and, of course, care assistants. Each member of this team plays a specific role, but all work towards a common goal: to promote the patient's functional and psychological recovery. This complementarity of skills is essential, as rehabilitation is not limited to a single dimension of care, but embraces the patient's body, mind and social environment.

Multi-disciplinary teamwork, which exists in other units, takes a different form here. In the rehabilitation department, the interdependence of interventions is crucial. Each member of the team relies on the observations and actions of the others to make the best possible adjustments to the care provided. For example, a physiotherapist can rely on the information provided by a caregiver on the evolution of a patient's mobility during daily care, while a psychologist can adapt his or her follow-up according to feedback from caregivers on the patient's mood or motivation. It is this fluidity of exchange and synergy of skills that makes the rehabilitation department so rich and special.

Another notable feature is that the pace and intensity of work differs from that observed in other medical units. Whereas acute care often requires urgent, intensive interventions over a short period of time, rehabilitation involves a long-term commitment. The patient's progress is sometimes slow, marked by advances and setbacks, and healthcare professionals, particularly nursing assistants, need to be both patient and persevering. This means accompanying patients at their own pace, supporting them psychologically in the face of their frustrations, and celebrating each small step forward with them. In this context, the temporality of care is not dictated by medical urgency, but by the patient's ability and receptiveness to rehabilitation.

The rehabilitation department is also distinguished by the nature of the care it provides. Where other units focus on technical interventions or pharmacological treatments, rehabilitation emphasizes care aimed at restoring lost or impaired functions. Hygiene and comfort care, for example, take on a much more therapeutic dimension here. The caregiver does more than simply wash or dress the patient; he or she gradually assists the patient in regaining his or her autonomy, encouraging him or her to actively participate in these daily gestures. Every action is designed not only to meet the patient's immediate needs, but also to enable him or her to regain motor or cognitive skills.

In addition, the atmosphere in the rehabilitation department is often characterized by close proximity and a closer relationship with patients, whether due to the prolonged duration of stays or the intensity of relational work. Patients, often faced with major functional losses, need constant psychological support, and this human dimension of care is central to the specific features of rehabilitation. The caregiver's constant presence becomes a familiar figure, a landmark in the sometimes difficult path of rehabilitation. This relationship of trust, which develops over time, is essential to maintaining the patient's motivation and encouraging him to persevere in his efforts, even when they seem fruitless.

Finally, the transition back home or to a specialized facility is a particularly important stage in the rehabilitation department, and represents another major difference from other units. Whereas most medical services focus on managing the acute phase of the disease, the rehabilitation service actively prepares the patient for reintegration into daily life, whether at home, in the workplace, or in an adapted structure. This involves constant assessment of the patient's ability to manage certain tasks independently, and education of the patient and family to ensure continuity of care in a less medicalized environment.

The different types of rehabilitation
  - Functional rehabilitation: neurological, orthopedic, cardiac, respiratory.

Functional rehabilitation is a complex and diversified field, tailored to the specific needs of each patient depending on the nature of the damage sustained. It spans several fields of specialization, including neurological, orthopedic, cardiac and respiratory rehabilitation. Each of these rehabilitations responds to particular challenges, depending on the body systems affected, but shares a common goal: to restore the patient's functional capabilities as far as possible, to enable him or her to regain optimal autonomy and quality of life.

In neurological rehabilitation, patients generally suffer from damage to the central or peripheral nervous system, resulting from stroke, head injury, multiple sclerosis or other neurological pathologies. These conditions often result in motor, sensory or cognitive deficits that impair the patient's ability to move, coordinate movements or perform everyday tasks. The neurological rehabilitation process revolves around the recovery of motor skills, coordination and muscular control. Physiotherapists play an essential role in relearning basic movements, such as walking or grasping, while occupational therapists help reorganize the patient's daily life, adapting the environment to his or her new abilities. The caregiver, for his part, accompanies the patient every step of the way, encouraging him during difficult moments, monitoring his progress and ensuring his safety, particularly during the first attempts at mobilization. In neurological rehabilitation, patience is key, as progress can be slow and fluctuating, but every small gain, every movement regained, is a significant victory for the patient and the care team.

Orthopedic rehabilitation focuses on patients who have undergone trauma or surgery affecting the musculoskeletal system: fractures, hip or knee replacements, amputations, or the aftermath of spinal surgery. The challenge here is to restore mobility and muscular strength, while ensuring the proper consolidation of bone and joint structures. In this context, rehabilitation exercises are often intensive, aimed at restoring range of motion, strengthening weakened muscles and relearning functional gestures such as standing up, walking or climbing stairs. The role of the caregiver is crucial here, particularly in preventing falls, supporting early mobilization and monitoring the onset of pain or complications such as post-operative infections or thrombosis. In collaboration with physiotherapists, the caregiver helps to keep the patient motivated, as orthopaedic rehabilitation can be physically demanding. But every step forward, whether it's improved knee flexion or a first step after surgery, is a step towards regaining autonomy.

Patients undergoing **cardiac rehabilitation** have often suffered a myocardial infarction, undergone heart surgery or are suffering from heart failure. The main aim of cardiac rehabilitation is to gradually build up cardiac capacity and improve exercise tolerance, while teaching the patient healthy lifestyle habits to prevent recurrence. Cardiac rehabilitation sessions include adapted physical exercises, under medical supervision, to re-train the heart to function efficiently while respecting its limits. The caregiver's role is to assist patients with these exercises, monitor their clinical condition (heart rate, blood pressure), and intervene rapidly in the event of signs of shortness of breath, chest pain or discomfort. The psychological dimension is also crucial: after a major cardiac event, patients often feel anxious or uncertain about their future abilities. The caregiver plays a supportive role in helping them regain confidence in their bodies, while ensuring that the efforts made remain within the safe limits defined by the medical team.

Finally, **respiratory rehabilitation** is aimed at patients suffering from chronic lung diseases, such as chronic obstructive pulmonary disease (COPD), severe asthma or after lung surgery. These conditions reduce lung capacity and exercise tolerance, making daily activities extremely demanding. The aim of rehabilitation is to improve respiratory efficiency and strengthen the muscles involved in breathing, through specific exercises, bronchial drainage techniques and adapted physical training. The nursing auxiliary plays a facilitating role, assisting patients with exercises, ensuring hydration and airway hygiene, and monitoring respiratory parameters. They are also responsible for reassuring patients, often distressed by their difficulty in breathing, by teaching them breathing techniques to manage breathlessness and accompanying them in their daily lives to reduce stress factors that aggravate symptoms.

- Post-trauma and post-surgical rehabilitation.

Post-traumatic and post-surgical rehabilitation plays a central role in the recovery process for patients who have suffered serious injuries or major surgery. These two types of rehabilitation share common goals: to help patients regain their functional abilities, restore their autonomy and, above all, enable them to reclaim their bodies after events that have profoundly altered them, whether an accident, a fracture, an amputation or a complex surgical operation. This process is essential to prevent the onset of complications and facilitate a return to everyday life under the best possible conditions.

Post-traumatic rehabilitation concerns people who have been victims of accidents or physical trauma, whether road accidents, falls, sports injuries or any other event that has caused fractures, sprains, muscle or nerve damage. In such cases, the body has been subjected to violent shocks which, in addition to physical damage, can have a lasting effect on the patient's confidence and perception of his or her own abilities. The aim of rehabilitation is twofold: to repair and to re-educate. Professionals, whether physiotherapists, occupational therapists or care assistants, work together to restore mobility, strength and functionality to injured limbs. But the psychological dimension is just as important, as trauma often leaves emotional scars that can hinder physical progress. The patient must learn to trust his or her body again, to overcome the fear of pain or recurrence, and sometimes to accept limitations that did not exist before the accident.

Post-traumatic rehabilitation usually begins with early mobilization, whenever the patient's condition permits. Once the acute phase is over, prolonged immobilization, although necessary for the healing of fractures or injuries, often leads to muscle wasting, loss of flexibility and reduced range of movement. Rehabilitation aims to counterbalance these effects by helping the patient gradually regain strength and mobility. This is achieved through adapted exercises, the use of technical aids and assistance in resuming the gestures of daily life. The caregiver plays a key role in this process, accompanying the patient during his or her first efforts, monitoring for signs of fatigue or pain, and encouraging the patient's active participation in his or her own rehabilitation.

In parallel, **post-surgical rehabilitation** takes place after an often heavy and intrusive operation, such as prosthesis fitting, orthopedic surgery (such as arthroplasty or ligament repair), or cardiac, thoracic or abdominal surgery. The aim here is to enable the body to recover not only from the surgery itself, but also from the effects of immobilization and anesthesia, which can lead to loss of muscle strength, joint stiffness and, sometimes, complications such as infections or respiratory disorders. Post-surgical rehabilitation often begins very early, sometimes even within the first few days after surgery, to prevent the onset of secondary complications such as pressure sores, venous thrombosis or scar adhesions.

The post-surgical rehabilitation process is organized around several axes. First, there is the management of post-operative pain, which can slow down mobilization. The caregiver, in collaboration with the medical team, ensures that pain is correctly assessed and treated, enabling the patient to actively participate in his or her rehabilitation. Then comes the gradual recovery of mobility, which depends on the type of operation. For orthopedic surgery, for example, gentle mobilization exercises are performed to prevent stiffening of the joints and keep the muscles supple. For more internal operations, such as cardiac or abdominal surgery, the emphasis is on respiratory rehabilitation, preventing pulmonary complications and regaining the ability to move without risk to the healing process.

One of the major challenges of post-traumatic and post-surgical rehabilitation lies in managing the patient's emotions and expectations. Many patients imagine that they will quickly regain their pre-accident or pre-surgery abilities, but the reality of the rehabilitation process is often slower and more complex. The caregiver, who is in direct daily contact with the patient, plays an essential role in providing moral support. They help to manage moments of frustration, encourage progress, however modest, and contribute to maintaining a positive attitude towards rehabilitation. This relationship of trust between patient and caregiver is crucial to the success of rehabilitation.

In some cases, post-traumatic or post-surgical rehabilitation may require long-term adaptations, especially if permanent sequelae remain. For example, a patient who has undergone amputation or partial paralysis will need to learn to use prostheses or technical aids, and to reorganize his or her activities of daily living in line with his or her new abilities. The support of the rehabilitation team, and in particular that of the caregivers, is crucial in helping the patient to navigate these new realities and develop strategies for living independently and satisfactorily.

Multidisciplinary teamwork

- The caregiver's place in the medical team: doctors, physiotherapists, occupational therapists.

The nursing auxiliary occupies an essential position within the medical team in the rehabilitation department, and its role is fundamental to the smooth running of the care process. Although their work is often seen as complementary to that of other healthcare professionals, the reality is that caregivers act as a key link in this multidisciplinary chain, seamlessly connecting the various players - doctors, physiotherapists and occupational therapists. Their daily, direct involvement with patients ensures continuity of care, while guaranteeing individualized, humane support.

The rehabilitation physician, at the heart of medical care, defines the patient's overall rehabilitation plan. He or she establishes a diagnosis, monitors clinical evolution and adjusts treatments according to progress made or complications encountered. However, he or she cannot be in constant contact with the patient. This is where the nursing auxiliary plays a crucial role. Present with patients on a daily basis, he or she is the watchful eye that observes small developments, signs of improvement or concern, and passes them on to the rest of the team. Thanks to their meticulous observation, orderlies help guide medical decisions by sharing often subtle but crucial information about the patient's physical or mental state. These precise, regular transmissions enable the doctor to adapt the care plan in a responsive, personalized way.

Furthermore, the nursing auxiliary is on the front line when it comes to applying and monitoring medical prescriptions, whether administering prescribed treatments or assisting with post-operative care, such as wound management, pain control or monitoring vital parameters. Their collaboration with the doctor is therefore not limited to the transmission of information: they actively contribute to the implementation of medical decisions, ensuring that care is adapted to the patient's condition on a day-to-day basis.

Collaboration with **physiotherapists** is also a central pillar of the nursing auxiliary's work. Physiotherapists' main task is to restore patients' mobility and muscle strength. They supervise rehabilitation sessions, define the exercises and guide the patient through the movements required to regain functional capacity. However, much of this rehabilitation continues outside the formal sessions. The caregiver's constant presence ensures that the instructions given by the physiotherapist are followed throughout the day. For example, they assist patients in their movements, helping them to carry out the recommended movements, while monitoring their posture and safety. He is also there to encourage patients to take an active part in their own rehabilitation, reminding them of the importance of every little effort made on a daily basis, whether transferring from bed to chair, or performing simple gestures such as getting up or walking.

In addition, caregivers play a vital role in **preventing complications** associated with immobility. When physiotherapists are not present, it is often the caregiver who ensures that the patient is properly installed in bed or in a chair, minimizing the risk of pressure sores or muscle atrophy. They also accompany patients during the initial phases of mobilization, providing physical support to prevent falls, while fostering confidence in their ability to move again.

As regards collaboration with **occupational therapists**, the nursing auxiliary plays a facilitating role in the rehabilitation of everyday movements. The occupational therapist helps the patient to relearn the essential actions of everyday life, such as dressing, washing or eating, taking into account the physical or cognitive limitations induced by the pathology. The caregiver extends this intervention by applying these principles to daily care. For example, they encourage patients to take an active part in their own grooming, helping them to use appropriate techniques to compensate for their limitations, or teaching them to use technical aids, such as grab bars or specialized tools to make it easier for them to hold objects.

The caregiver is often the one who accompanies the patient in repeating these gestures throughout the day, outside the sessions with the occupational therapist. In this way, they reinforce the patient's autonomy, while adjusting their support according to the patient's actual abilities and state of fatigue. This ongoing involvement ensures steady progress, as every daily gesture, however trivial, becomes an opportunity to learn or relearn.

On a relational level, the nursing auxiliary brings a human dimension that complements that of other team members. By being close to the patient on a daily basis, they are often the first to perceive any emotional or psychological difficulties that the patient may encounter during rehabilitation. This proximity enables the caregiver to play a moral support role, comforting the patient at times of doubt or discouragement. In this way, the caregiver facilitates the patient's adherence to the rehabilitation program, helping him or her to overcome the fears and frustrations associated with physical limitations.

- Interactions with patients and families.

Interaction with patients and their families plays a central role in the caregiver's day-to-day work, particularly in the rehabilitation department, where support is not limited to physical care, but extends to emotional support and listening to patients' deepest needs. Rehabilitation, which is often long and demanding, requires a relationship of trust and fluid communication between patients, their families and the entire care team. The caregiver, through his or her constant presence and role as first point of contact, becomes the essential link in this dynamic, transmitting information, listening to concerns and managing expectations.

The relationship with the patient goes far beyond simply providing care. The caregiver is the person who, day after day, accompanies the patient on his or her rehabilitation journey, supporting them during moments of doubt and encouraging them in the face of even the slightest progress. This proximity enables the caregiver to understand the patient's individual needs, whether physical or psychological. Every care gesture becomes an opportunity to create a bond, to reassure and motivate. For example, during hygiene care, which can be a vulnerable time for the patient, the caregiver establishes a relationship of respect and dignity, enabling the patient to feel cared for in a human and attentive way. This attention to detail, such as the way a patient prefers to be helped, or his or her small victories in daily life, helps to build a lasting relationship of trust.

The psychological dimension of this interaction is particularly important in a context where many patients may experience feelings of frustration, helplessness and even depression. Temporary or permanent loss of autonomy is a major upheaval in the life of any individual, and the caregiver is often in the front line to perceive these moments of distress. By actively listening to the emotions and fears expressed, the caregiver can play a role of moral support, enabling the patient to feel understood and encouraged. This dimension of empathy, even in brief exchanges, helps to create an environment conducive to rehabilitation, where the patient feels supported not only in his physical recovery, but also in his mental struggle against the fear of not regaining his abilities.

Interaction is not limited to the patient. The **family**, often anxious and sometimes helpless in the face of their loved one's situation, also plays an important role in the rehabilitation process, and the caregiver must know how to manage this relationship with tact and professionalism. Relatives are often the people who know the patient best, and who will be the main support once the patient has been discharged. It is therefore crucial to involve them in the process, while providing them with the necessary information on the progress of rehabilitation and the patient's needs. The caregiver then becomes an essential mediator between the medical team and the family, explaining in a clear and accessible way the progress made, the exercises to be continued, or the care to be anticipated once the patient has returned home.

Interacting with families requires a great deal of listening and teaching skills. Relatives, in the throes of uncertainty or worry, often seek to understand what their loved ones are going through, and what they can do to help. The caregiver plays a fundamental role in explaining the rehabilitation process, clarifying realistic expectations and answering questions sympathetically. Sometimes, this also means allaying excessive worries, while giving practical advice on what to do to help the patient through rehabilitation. The caregiver must then ensure that family members feel supported, informed and involved, without being overwhelmed by responsibilities they may not feel able to take on.

What's more, the return home or to an adapted facility is often a complex stage to prepare, both for the patient and the family. The caregiver contributes to this preparation by providing concrete recommendations and ensuring that the family understands the patient's specific needs: how to accompany him/her in his/her movements, what exercises to encourage, what precautions to take to avoid falls or other complications. This preparation helps reduce the anxiety of loved ones, while giving them the tools they need to play an active role in the continuity of care at home.

In some cases, families may also find themselves faced with emotional dilemmas, particularly when the patient's progress is slow or permanent after-effects complicate the return to a normal life. As the care team's intermediary, the caregiver needs to be sensitive when broaching these subjects with the family, taking care not to raise false hopes while encouraging a positive, realistic approach. Managing the emotions of both the patient and his or her loved ones is a key aspect of support, and the caregiver is often the one who, by being close to them on a daily basis, helps to maintain a balance between hope and pragmatism.

The specific missions of the rehabilitation orderly
- Ensure the well-being and clinical monitoring of patients.

Ensuring the well-being and clinical monitoring of patients is one of the fundamental missions of the caregiver, particularly in rehabilitation, where meticulous monitoring of the patient's physical and psychological state is essential to guarantee optimum recovery. This dual role, both preventive and curative, relies on constant attention to the patient's needs and heightened vigilance regarding his state of health, in order to detect the slightest signs of complication or improvement. This monitoring, although it may seem routine, is in fact crucial, as it enables care to be rapidly adjusted to subtle changes in the patient's condition.

A patient's well-being depends first and foremost on the quality of the care provided on a daily basis. In rehabilitation, physical comfort is of prime importance, as it often determines the patient's active participation in his or her own recovery. The caregiver ensures that the patient is positioned appropriately, avoiding prolonged postures that could lead to pain, pressure sores or respiratory discomfort. This attention to detail, such as adjusting pillows, regularly repositioning the patient or providing support when moving around, contributes directly to improving the patient's quality of life during their stay. By taking care of every aspect of comfort, the caregiver creates an environment conducive to recovery, where the patient feels supported and respected in his or her needs.

Wellness is more than just physical care. It also encompasses a psychological dimension that is just as important in the rehabilitation process. Rehabilitation patients, often faced with a temporary or permanent loss of autonomy, may experience feelings of frustration, discouragement or fear about the future. The caregiver, through his or her daily presence and direct contact with the patient, plays a key role in providing moral support and establishing a climate of trust. By listening to patients' concerns, answering their questions and reassuring them of the progress they are making, the caregiver helps to reduce anxiety and reinforce patients' motivation to take an active part in their rehabilitation.

Clinical monitoring, on the other hand, is a more technical but equally crucial aspect of the nursing auxiliary's work. It involves careful, continuous observation of the patient's vital signs and reactions to the care provided. Every day, the caregiver checks parameters such as the patient's body temperature, pulse, blood pressure and breathing. This information, gathered on a regular basis, is used to monitor the patient's state of health and detect any signs of deterioration. For example, a rise in temperature may indicate the onset of an infection, while irregular breathing may signal a respiratory complication. These observations, often made outside examination times by the doctor or nurses, are vital for rapid intervention in the event of a problem.

The caregiver must also be alert to less obvious but equally important signs, such as skin color, the presence of edema or redness, or the patient's expressions of pain. Some patients, particularly those with cognitive or communication difficulties, may not be able to verbally express their pain or discomfort. This is where the caregiver's experience and intuition come into play. By carefully observing the patient's behavior, noting changes in posture, appetite or sleep, the caregiver can spot subtle signs of discomfort or suffering. These observations, though often discreet, are of vital importance in preventing more serious complications.

At the same time, clinical monitoring also requires heightened vigilance during rehabilitation activities. When mobilizing patients, for example, the caregiver must be attentive to the patient's physical reactions during and after the effort. Excessive fatigue, intense pain or dizziness may be signs that the patient is exceeding his or her limits, necessitating adjustment of the exercises or reassessment by the medical team. This constant vigilance helps avoid the risk of falls or accidents, while ensuring progressive rehabilitation adapted to the patient's abilities.

Pressure sore prevention is another key aspect of clinical monitoring. Bedridden patients or those with reduced mobility are particularly vulnerable to pressure sores, skin lesions that form as a result of prolonged pressure on certain parts of the body. The caregiver must regularly reposition the patient to relieve these pressure areas, while carefully monitoring the condition of the skin. They play a key preventive role by applying specific care protocols, such as the use of decubitus-anti cushions or mattresses, and moisturizing the patient's skin to preserve its integrity.

Finally, the preventive aspect of the caregiver's role also extends to pain management. By monitoring the patient's expressions and signs of pain, the caregiver can adjust his or her approach to make care less uncomfortable, while alerting the medical team when additional pain relief treatments are required. This careful monitoring ensures that the patient does not suffer unnecessarily, while encouraging more active participation in rehabilitation, as a patient relieved of pain is a patient more willing to engage in rehabilitation exercises.

- Facilitate patients' rehabilitation and reintegration into everyday life.

Facilitating patients' rehabilitation and reintegration into everyday life is one of the most fundamental and rewarding missions of the rehabilitation department. This involves guiding patients through a complex process in which, after experiencing illness, trauma or surgery, they must relearn to perform essential actions, regain their autonomy and resume their place in society. This process is not limited to simple physical rehabilitation; it encompasses comprehensive work that integrates the patient's body, mind and environment, to enable a gradual but complete return to a functional and fulfilling life.

Rehabilitation starts with restoring the patient's physical capabilities. After an accident or surgery, many patients find themselves confronted with limitations they've never experienced before: difficulty walking, using their hands, standing upright, or even performing tasks as simple as getting up from a chair or picking up an object. It is at this stage that the caregiver, in collaboration with physiotherapists and occupational therapists, plays a key role. It's not just a question of physically assisting the patient to carry out these movements, but also of restoring his or her confidence in his or her abilities. Every gesture, however simple, must be encouraged and repeated, so that the patient progresses and strengthens his or her motor skills. The caregiver ensures that these movements become increasingly autonomous, by providing the necessary support without doing things for the patient. For example, when washing or eating, the caregiver's role is to support the patient in these daily gestures, while encouraging him or her to carry them out on their own, even if only partially.

Physical rehabilitation goes hand in hand with constant moral support. Loss of autonomy, whether temporary or permanent, can lead to profound self-questioning, frustration and even psychological distress. The caregiver is often the one who, through his or her daily presence and active listening, soothes these anxieties. He or she motivates the patient to continue with rehabilitation exercises, even when progress seems slow or difficult. This close relationship helps patients to feel supported in their efforts to relearn, while strengthening their will to overcome the challenges they face. Re-education, although physical in its approach, is also a psychological process that requires strong resilience. The caregiver, by listening to the patient's frustrations and doubts, plays a crucial role in maintaining positive morale throughout this period.

Once physical progress has been made, the next stage in rehabilitation is the patient's gradual reintegration into everyday life. This involves adapting the movements learned during rehabilitation sessions to the reality of everyday life. It's not enough to be able to stand up or walk a few steps in the rehabilitation room; the real objective is to enable the patient to return to a lifestyle that is as independent as possible, whether at home, at work or in the community. The caregiver plays an essential role here. For example, they help the patient to relearn practical gestures, such as cooking, dressing, going up and down stairs, or managing everyday objects. Each re-education exercise is geared towards a return to reality, so that the patient can gradually reintegrate these gestures into his or her daily life.

Rehabilitation also requires special attention to the patient's specific needs and environment. Sometimes, rehabilitation must be accompanied by adaptation of the living environment or the use of technical aids. The caregiver, in collaboration with the occupational therapist, assists the patient in using these aids, such as walkers, grab bars or wheelchairs. They ensure that the patient knows how to use these aids independently, while guaranteeing their safety. This learning phase is crucial to avoid the risk of falls or injury, while promoting the patient's autonomy in the home environment.

Support for patient reintegration also extends to the involvement of family and friends. Returning home after a long period of hospitalization or rehabilitation can be a source of anxiety for patients, especially when they have not fully recovered. The caregiver, in conjunction with the multidisciplinary team, prepares for this transition by informing and educating family and friends about how to support the patient in daily life. The aim is not only to teach them how to help the patient physically, but also to provide them with the tools to support him morally and encourage him to maintain his achievements. By explaining the patient's specific needs and strategies for avoiding complications, the caregiver plays a crucial role in the success of home reintegration.

Finally, for some patients, reintegration also involves a gradual return to the world of work or social activities. This step is essential to restore meaning to the patient's life and boost his or her self-esteem. The caregiver, in collaboration with social workers and occupational therapists, contributes to this reintegration by helping the patient regain confidence in his or her ability to evolve in an external environment. This may involve simple outings, the resumption of social habits, or the consideration of a professional activity adapted to the patient's new abilities. This aspect of reintegration is often the culmination of the rehabilitation process, as it symbolizes the patient's return to a more independent and active life.

Chapter 2

Welcoming and assessing the patient: The crucial observation stage

Reception in the rehabilitation department: A key moment

- Care on arrival: listening and humanity.

Taking care of a patient on arrival in a rehabilitation department is a crucial stage, often determining the course of his or her entire course of care. It's a delicate moment when patients, often weakened by illness, surgery or accident, arrive in a new environment, far removed from their familiar surroundings and sometimes fraught with uncertainty. Right from the start, the caregiver's ability to listen attentively and show humanity is essential to creating a climate of trust and calming the patient's anxieties. These qualities, which form the basis of a successful care relationship, help not only to establish a respectful rapport, but also to lay the foundations for effective, caring support throughout the rehabilitation process.

When a patient walks through the doors of a rehabilitation department, he or she usually arrives in a vulnerable state. Physically, they may be weakened, limited in their movements, or suffering from residual pain. Psychologically, they may be troubled by uncertainty about their ability to recover, or by fear of losing their autonomy for good. The caregiver, who is often one of the patient's first contacts, must be particularly sensitive to this fragility. An active listening attitude from the outset helps to reassure the patient and answer his or her initial questions. By taking the time to let the patient express his or her concerns and expectations, as well as his or her doubts, the caregiver shows that he or she is there to provide personalized support, in an approach that goes beyond the simple provision of technical care.

Humanity, in these first moments, translates into small attentions that seem insignificant, but are essential to the patient's well-being. These are simple gestures: smiling, asking open-ended questions, using a soothing tone of voice, introducing yourself with kindness, while explaining to the patient what is going to happen in the hours and days ahead. These actions help reduce the stress that patients can feel when they find themselves in a hospital setting, often perceived as impersonal or intimidating. It's these caring gestures that make patients feel seen and heard as individuals, not reduced to pathologies or file numbers.

This initial care is not limited to listening to the patient's medical needs, but takes into account the whole person. Rehabilitation patients often have questions that go beyond the strict framework of care: concerns about their daily life, their family, their future. The caregiver's open, empathetic attitude can capture these questions and respond appropriately, or direct the patient to the appropriate professionals, such as social workers or psychologists. Establishing an open dialogue from the outset helps patients to understand that they will be supported not only physically, but also emotionally and socially, in a holistic and humane approach.

In addition to listening and showing humanity, care on arrival also involves a certain amount of teaching. When patients arrive in a rehabilitation department, they need to understand what awaits them. The nursing auxiliary has an important educational role here: it explains the different stages of the rehabilitation process, how the department works, and the rules to be followed to ensure optimal care. This transparency helps patients to feel secure and to know what to expect. When care and objectives are clearly explained, patients become more active players in their rehabilitation, as they better understand the reasons for the care they are receiving.

Care is not only provided on an individual basis, but also involves the patient's family whenever possible. Relatives are often worried or disoriented about their parent's or partner's situation, and need to be reassured and informed. By taking the time to welcome the family as well, the caregiver helps to create a serene environment conducive to rehabilitation. This interaction helps to reinforce the support the patient will receive outside the hospital, by explaining to relatives how they can accompany him/her, preparing them for certain aspects of the care pathway, and answering their questions. This helps to integrate rehabilitation into the patient's daily life once he or she has returned home.

Finally, humanity in initial care also means adapting to the specific needs and expectations of each patient. It's essential to recognize that every person is unique, and that every rehabilitation journey will be different. Some patients may be impatient to start rehabilitation, while others may be more reluctant, frightened by the pain or effort involved. The caregiver needs to know how to adapt his or her approach, listening to these signals, and adjusting the level of support and encouragement needed. Sometimes, this means taking the time to talk at greater length with a patient who is expressing fears, or on the contrary, firmly supporting those who are in a greater hurry to make progress but need to be tempered to avoid relapses or over-exertion.

- Creating a safe, reassuring environment.

Creating a safe and reassuring environment is a fundamental aspect of working in a rehabilitation department. For patients who are often emerging from an acute phase of care, or recovering from physical or psychological trauma, feeling safe and secure is vital to their recovery. Such an environment is not just about physical safety, but also about emotional well-being. It is in this safe space, where patients know they can progress without risk, that they find the confidence they need to re-engage in their rehabilitation and, ultimately, regain their autonomy. Caregivers play a key role in building this climate of security, through their constant attention, the quality of the care they provide and the relationship of trust they establish with the patient.

First and foremost, physical safety is based on preventing the risks associated with patients' loss of mobility or physical weaknesses. Many of those arriving for rehabilitation have reduced mobility, are prone to falls, or suffer from post-operative pain, joint stiffness or dizziness. The caregiver must be constantly vigilant to the patient's condition, adapting care and facilities to prevent any incidents. For example, the caregiver ensures the correct use of support devices, such as grab bars, walkers or wheelchairs, to ensure that every move is made safely. They must also ensure that the patient's bed is adjusted to the right height, that passageways are clear and that technical aids are always within reach, so that the patient does not take unnecessary risks by trying to move around unaided.

At the same time, the caregiver plays a preventive role, closely monitoring the patient for signs of fatigue or pain. They ensure that rehabilitation exercises, while necessary, do not exceed the patient's capabilities, to avoid injury or worsening of symptoms. This constant vigilance maintains a balance between the effort required and safety, encouraging smooth progress towards independence. By doing so, the caregiver gives the patient the certainty that he or she can work on rehabilitation in a setting where every gesture is monitored, every step is controlled, and risks are minimized.

Secondly, creating a reassuring environment means establishing a relationship of trust between the patient and the care team. The caregiver, through his or her daily contact, is often the person who embodies this closeness. This relationship relies on the active listening and availability of the caregiver, who must be able to perceive the patient's unexpressed needs and respond to their concerns. A patient undergoing rehabilitation can feel vulnerable, particularly when he or she has to relearn how to perform basic movements that were previously performed without effort. The caring presence of the caregiver, who encourages without rushing, helps the patient to overcome his or her fears. He knows that, even if he stumbles, he will be supported. This reassurance is crucial for daring to undertake exercises or movements that may seem frightening after long immobilization or a complex operation.

The caregiver's humanity and understanding in daily interactions also contribute to creating a psychologically reassuring environment. Patients, often faced with uncertainty about their future, may express doubts about their ability to recover or regain their autonomy. The caregiver's moral support, availability and empathetic attitude help to dispel these anxieties. Every little bit of progress is valued, every worry taken seriously. In this way, the patient feels not only physically safe, but also emotionally supported, enabling him or her to make more serene progress in rehabilitation.

The familiarity and consistency of the caregiver's care also play a fundamental role in the patient's sense of security. The daily routine of care, whether hygiene, meals or rehabilitation, is in itself a factor of stability. For a patient who has often experienced a sudden break in his or her life due to illness or accident, these regular, routine gestures provide a predictable, structuring framework. By ensuring continuity of care, the caregiver enables the patient to find his or her bearings over time, and gradually regain control over his or her body and daily life. This consistency of care also enables patients to anticipate the stages of their rehabilitation, reinforcing their sense of control and security.

Finally, the reassuring dimension of a rehabilitation environment is not only for the patient, but also for his or her loved ones. Families, who are often worried about their loved one's state of health, find reassurance in knowing that the patient is being cared for in a safe, caring environment. The caregiver, by communicating regularly with the family, explaining the care provided and the progress made, contributes to this peace of mind. When the family is reassured, they themselves become a support to the patient, further fostering an overall environment of trust and security.

Day-to-day clinical observation
  ○   Recognize signs of improvement or complications. Recognizing signs of improvement or complications in a patient undergoing rehabilitation is a crucial task, requiring the caregiver to observe carefully and be sensitive to the slightest physical,

emotional or behavioral changes. Rehabilitation is a long and often complex process, where progress can be slow and complications sometimes insidious. By being in daily contact with the patient, the caregiver is particularly well placed to spot these developments, whether positive or negative, and to inform the medical team in order to adjust management. This vigilance is essential not only to maximize the patient's chances of recovery, but also to prevent complications that could compromise progress.

Signs of improvement can take many forms and appear gradually. Physically, they often take the form of increased mobility or muscle strength, better coordination of movements, or greater autonomy in everyday activities. A patient who can get up unaided, walk longer without assistance, or perform simple tasks such as dressing or bathing, is showing concrete signs of recovery. By accompanying the patient in these activities, the caregiver can not only observe this progress, but also encourage it. He or she is often the first to notice that the patient needs less assistance, tires less quickly or seems more confident in his or her movements. These small but subtle signs are valuable indicators that rehabilitation is moving in the right direction.

Improvement can also be seen in reduced pain or better symptom management. A patient who complains of less pain, is able to breathe better after respiratory rehabilitation, or is more at ease with physical activities, often signals good progress. The caregiver, by listening to these changes and carefully monitoring the patient's reactions during care or exercise, is able to spot these improvements, however small. This enables the care team to measure the effectiveness of treatments and to continue to adapt care in the best possible way.

Beyond the physical aspects, signs of improvement can also be seen on a psychological level. A rehabilitation patient who begins to regain self-confidence, expresses greater motivation or shows enthusiasm for his or her rehabilitation is a patient on the road to recovery. The caregiver, through his or her proximity and constant support, is well placed to pick up on these changes in attitude. A smile, positive speech, an increased desire to take part in exercises or daily activities are all encouraging signs that the patient is regaining confidence in his or her abilities. The caregiver plays a crucial role here, not only in observing these improvements, but also in reinforcing them by encouraging the patient, congratulating him on his efforts and motivating him to continue.

However, recognizing the **signs of complications** is just as important. Rehabilitation can be marked by periods of stagnation or regression, which require special attention. Physical complications can manifest themselves in different ways, such as increased pain, greater difficulty in performing previously acquired movements, or the appearance of new symptoms, such as edema, redness, pressure sores or infection. For example, a patient who complains of new or increased pain after exertion may be signalling inflammation or another underlying problem. By observing these changes and asking targeted questions, the caregiver can identify these signs at an early stage and quickly alert the medical team.

Complications can also take the form of a general deterioration in the patient's state of health. Excessive fatigue, loss of appetite, changes in behavior or difficulty in breathing are all warning signs that need to be taken very seriously. The caregiver, who knows the patient well, is often able to spot these subtle changes even before the patient expresses them. For example, a patient who was able to walk a short distance but suddenly shows signs of shortness of breath or increased weakness could have developed a complication, such as a lung infection or heart problem. These signals, however discreet, must be communicated immediately to the rest of the team for a thorough medical assessment.

Complications are not just physical. Psychologically, a patient undergoing rehabilitation can sometimes show signs of depression, discouragement or anxiety. Although less visible, these signs can have a major impact on the patient's progress. An apathetic attitude, loss of interest in exercise or care, repeated complaints of fatigue or increasing isolation are indicators that the patient is experiencing emotional or mental difficulties. By listening and supporting the patient, the caregiver can pick up on these signals and bring them to the attention of the care team, in order to offer psychological support or adjust the rehabilitation plan according to the patient's mental state. Ignoring these signs could slow down rehabilitation or worsen the patient's condition.

The caregiver's ability to recognize signs of improvement or complications relies on constant vigilance and a good knowledge of the patient. By being present on a daily basis and building a relationship of trust with the patient, the caregiver is able to detect subtle changes that may go unnoticed by other team members. His observations, which he passes on at care meetings or in written transmissions, are a valuable source of information for adjusting treatments and rehabilitation exercises in real time.

- Tools for monitoring and communicating with the care team.

Tools for monitoring and communicating with the care team are essential elements in the management of rehabilitation patients. They ensure smooth coordination between the various healthcare professionals, provide constant, precise monitoring of patient progress, and enable rapid reaction to any complications. In a rehabilitation department, where progress can be slow and signs of improvement or regression subtle, these tools are crucial for adjusting care and optimizing the rehabilitation pathway. As the professional in direct and regular contact with the patient, the caregiver plays a key role in the use of these tools, as he or she is often the first to notice small changes in the patient's state of health.

Clinical monitoring relies on simple but essential tools, which enable the evolution of the patient's vital parameters to be followed in real time. Among the most common are temperature, blood pressure, pulse, respiratory rate and sometimes oxygen saturation. These measurements, taken on a regular basis, provide valuable information on the patient's state of health. A sudden change, such as a rise in temperature, a change in blood pressure or unusual shortness of breath, can be a sign of complication and requires rapid intervention by the medical team. The caregiver, through constant observation, must not only record these data, but also be able to interpret them sufficiently to alert other team members if necessary.

In addition to these physical parameters, caregivers also use **evaluation scales** to assess the patient's pain, mobility and autonomy. For example, the Visual Analog Scale (VAS) is a simple but effective tool for measuring the pain felt by the patient. By asking the patient to rate his or her pain on a scale of 1 to 10, the caregiver can adapt care accordingly. Similarly, specific scales, such as the Braden scale to assess the risk of pressure sores, or the Borg scale to measure the perception of effort during physical rehabilitation, enable care to be adjusted to the patient's specific needs. These seemingly simple tools are essential for fine-tuned monitoring of the patient's state of health, and for preventing the onset of complications.

Behavioral observation is another valuable tool in clinical monitoring. Through regular contact with the patient, the caregiver is often the first to notice subtle changes in the patient's behavior or emotional state. Unusual fatigue, lack of motivation, gradual isolation or a drop in appetite can be warning signs of physical or psychological complications. These observations, although not always reflected in figures or measurements, are just as important for the overall management of the patient. By remaining attentive to these signals, the caregiver can pass them on to the care team so that adjustments can be made, whether in treatment, rehabilitation or psychological support.

One of the most fundamental communication tools is **written transmission**, in the form of care records or targeted transmissions. At each change of service or end of shift, the orderly records the observations made during the day in the patient's file. They record vital parameters, the care provided, the patient's reactions and their observations of the patient's general condition. This file, shared with the entire care team, is an essential database for ensuring continuity of care. It enables a precise record to be kept of the patient's progress, and any improvements or complications to be monitored day by day. By recording observations clearly and in detail, the nursing auxiliary ensures that every member of the team has the information they need to adapt their care.

At the same time, **team meetings** are another essential communication tool. They enable the various members of the multi-disciplinary team - doctors, nurses, physiotherapists, occupational therapists and care assistants - to get together to discuss the patient's progress. The caregiver, through his or her direct daily contact with the patient, makes a valuable contribution to these meetings. He or she can share specific details of how the patient is responding to care, rehabilitation exercises or the environment. For example, he or she may report an improvement in the patient's ability to walk, a reduction in pain levels or, conversely, increasing difficulty in certain activities. This regular, structured communication enables us to implement appropriate strategies and ensure consistency in the care provided by each member of the team.

Digital tools, increasingly present in healthcare establishments, also facilitate monitoring and communication. Computerized medical records centralize all patient information, accessible to the entire healthcare team in real time. These systems make it possible to record not only clinical observations, but also treatments administered, test results, and even instructions from the multidisciplinary team. By accessing these digital tools, the caregiver can consult the patient's latest medical data and update daily care information in real time. This ensures a fluid flow of information and greater responsiveness to any changes in the patient's condition.

Verbal communication remains an indispensable tool, especially in times of emergency or sudden change in the patient's condition. When a problem is detected - such as acute pain, a fall or a respiratory problem - the caregiver must be able to pass on his or her observations immediately to the nurse or doctor on duty. This rapid communication enables immediate intervention and reduces the risk of serious complications. Similarly, when changing shifts, care assistants pass on the information essential for continuity of care, so that nothing is overlooked in the management of the patient.

The caregiver's role in assessing patient autonomy
  ○   Autonomy evaluation grids and their use.

Autonomy evaluation grids play a crucial role in the care of rehabilitation patients, as they enable precise measurement of their ability to perform the essential gestures of daily life. These tools are essential for assessing patient progress over time, adapting care and rehabilitation exercises, and identifying specific needs in terms of assistance. The caregiver, who accompanies the patient on a day-to-day basis, is at the heart of the use of these grids, as he or she is in direct contact with concrete situations where the patient's autonomy is put to the test. These assessments are essential not only for drawing up an appropriate care plan, but also for monitoring the patient's progress, adjusting rehabilitation objectives and promoting a gradual return to independence.

Autonomy evaluation grids are used to assess a patient's functions and abilities in a variety of areas, such as mobility, hygiene, eating, dressing and transferring (from bed to chair, from sitting to standing, etc.). Each area of daily life is carefully scrutinized, and the patient is assessed according to criteria that measure his or her degree of independence: can he or she perform certain tasks alone? Does he need partial or total assistance? The answers to these questions enable us to determine the level of assistance required, and to implement targeted actions to improve autonomy.

One of the most frequently used grids in this context is the **Barthel index**, which measures a patient's ability to perform 10 activities of daily living, such as eating, washing, getting around or using the toilet. Each activity is scored according to the patient's degree of autonomy, and the scores are added together to establish an overall index of dependence or independence. For example, a patient who is totally autonomous in dressing or bathing will obtain a maximum score in these areas, while a patient who requires complete assistance will see his or her score reduced. This grid is particularly useful, as it provides an overview of the patient's needs and enables realistic, personalized rehabilitation objectives to be set.

In using these grids, the caregiver plays a fundamental role. By being present during daily care, he or she is able to observe the patient's behavior and see how he or she reacts in real-life situations. When the patient tries to get up on his own, eat or wash, the caregiver can note the difficulties encountered, how the patient adapts, or whether he shows signs of improvement. These observations are then translated into objective data, using the grid to quantify the patient's progress or regression.

The use of evaluation grids is not limited to simply collecting data. They are also a valuable tool for **adapting care**. For example, if the grid reveals that the patient is having increasing difficulty transferring alone, the rehabilitation team may decide to intensify mobility exercises or provide technical aids, such as grab bars or an adapted wheelchair. Conversely, if the grid shows a gradual improvement in mobility, this may be a signal to encourage the patient to move around more independently, while gradually reducing the level of assistance.

These grids are also essential for **monitoring** patient **progress** over the long term. In fact, they enable us to measure progress or stagnation from one day to the next, or from one week to the next, and to see whether the objectives set have been achieved. By regularly recording the results of assessments, caregivers provide the medical and paramedical team with precise information to help them adjust rehabilitation programs. If a patient is progressing faster than expected in certain tasks, the grid can be used to redefine objectives for further rehabilitation. If, on the contrary, blockages appear, the grid can be used to reassess priorities and focus on problem areas.

Another advantage of autonomy evaluation grids is that they **encourage patients to take an active role in their rehabilitation**. In fact, by regularly measuring their abilities, patients can see the progress they are making, even if it is sometimes slow or modest. These tools make visible improvements that may go unnoticed on a day-to-day basis, such as increased muscle strength, improved coordination or greater mobility. Seeing these progress figures encourages patients to continue their efforts, because they know that every exercise, every gesture counts in the rehabilitation process. It also boosts motivation and involvement, making patients feel more responsible for their own progress.

Finally, autonomy evaluation grids are **effective communication** tools within the care team. The data collected by caregivers during daily care is shared with nurses, rehabilitation physicians, physiotherapists and occupational therapists, giving everyone a clear, objective view of the patient's needs. This fluid communication is essential for adjusting care and avoiding mistakes, such as over-assistance that could hinder the patient's autonomy, or on the contrary a lack of support in situations where the patient still needs it. By centralizing information on the patient's state of autonomy, these grids facilitate informed, coordinated decision-making within the multidisciplinary team.

- Participate in adjusting the care plan according to the patient's progress.

Participating in the adjustment of the care plan according to the patient's progress is one of the essential missions of the care assistant in the rehabilitation department. This role, which goes far beyond the provision of basic care, is based on close, ongoing observation of the patient's physical and psychological condition, and on close collaboration with the medical and paramedical team. The aim is to adapt care and interventions according to the patient's progress, needs and sometimes regression, in order to optimize his or her rehabilitation pathway and facilitate his or her return to independence.

Rehabilitation is a dynamic process, where each day can bring subtle or significant changes in the patient's state of health. The caregiver, through his or her daily presence and direct contact with the patient, is often the first to detect these changes, whether positive or negative. For example, they may observe a gradual improvement in the patient's mobility, a reduction in pain, or, on the contrary, the appearance of new difficulties, such as increased fatigue, more intense pain, or signs of discouragement. These observations, although sometimes discreet, are essential for adjusting the care plan so that it remains relevant and effective.

When the caregiver notices **progress** in the patient's condition, he or she may suggest, in consultation with the care team, adjusting the level of assistance provided. For example, a patient who is able to get up unaided with greater ease, or to walk a longer distance, may require less physical support, allowing greater autonomy. By relaying this information during transmissions or team meetings, the caregiver helps to adapt rehabilitation objectives and encourage a more independence-oriented approach. This type of adjustment is crucial to avoid over-assistance, which could slow down rehabilitation by keeping the patient in a state of unnecessary dependence.

Conversely, if the caregiver observes **increasing difficulties** or signs of regression, it is equally important to reassess the care plan. A patient showing unusual fatigue, new pain or loss of interest in activities may need extra support. These signs may indicate that the pace of rehabilitation is too intense, or that complications are developing. In such cases, the caregiver plays an alert role by reporting these changes to the medical team, enabling rehabilitation exercises to be adjusted, pain relief treatments to be reviewed or additional technical aids to be put in place to facilitate the patient's movements. This adaptation process prevents patient exhaustion and maintains a balance between the efforts required and the patient's actual capabilities at any given time.

Adjusting the care plan is not limited to physical aspects alone. The patient's psychological state plays a central role in his or her rehabilitation, and the caregiver, by listening to the patient's emotions and concerns, also contributes to the adjustment of the psychological support provided. A patient who shows signs of discouragement or frustration at progress deemed too slow may benefit from reinforced moral support, or from a reorganization of rehabilitation sessions to make them less restrictive. By showing empathy and understanding, the caregiver can suggest adaptations that make rehabilitation more accessible and less stressful for the patient, while encouraging his or her commitment to the process.

Teamwork is at the heart of this adjustment process. The caregiver's observations are invaluable, as they provide concrete information on how the patient is reacting on a daily basis. During written or verbal transmissions, as well as during multidisciplinary meetings, the caregiver shares his or her observations on the patient's progress, giving nurses, rehabilitation physicians, physiotherapists and occupational therapists an overview of the situation. For example, if a patient is progressing faster than expected in certain areas, this may lead to a revision of the rehabilitation objectives, by increasing the complexity of the exercises or diversifying the proposed activities. Conversely, if unforeseen difficulties arise, such as pain that limits mobility, the care plan can be temporarily lightened to allow the patient to recover without jeopardizing the progress made.

Another important aspect of adjusting the care plan is **preventing complications**. Through careful observation, the caregiver is often the first to spot warning signs of complications, such as the appearance of redness or bedsores in bedridden patients, signs of infection, or respiratory problems in cardiac or pulmonary rehabilitation patients. By alerting the care team to these signs at an early stage, it enables them to react proactively, adjusting the care plan to prevent the situation worsening. This may include changes in the frequency of hygiene care, the use of pressure sore prevention equipment, or the implementation of new respiratory rehabilitation strategies.

Adjusting the care plan also means **regularly reassessing** rehabilitation **objectives** in line with the patient's progress. If a patient achieves certain objectives more quickly than expected, such as autonomy in transfers or the ability to feed oneself, the care team, with input from the caregiver, may decide to raise the objectives or introduce new activities to further stimulate the patient's abilities. On the other hand, if the initial objectives prove too ambitious, it is essential to scale them down, so as not to discourage the patient or risk overloading his or her body and mind. The caregiver, being in constant contact with the patient, is a key player in this reassessment, as he or she is the one who knows best the patient's current limits and potential capacities.

Chapter 3

Supporting basic care in a rehabilitation context

Hygiene care for rehabilitation patients
- Body hygiene: adapting care to physical limitations.

Personal hygiene is an essential dimension of patient care, particularly in rehabilitation, where physical limitations require constant adaptation of gestures and techniques. For a patient with temporary or permanent loss of mobility, hygiene care is not just a matter of comfort, but plays a key role in preventing medical complications, while helping to preserve the patient's dignity and psychological well-being. As the person responsible for this care, the caregiver must adapt his or her approach to the patient's physical capabilities, while encouraging autonomy wherever possible. This adaptation requires both close attention to the specific needs of each patient, and a mastery of the techniques needed to guarantee respectful and effective care, without jeopardizing patient safety.

One of the first steps in adapting personal hygiene care is to **assess** the patient's **physical capabilities**. Some patients may be able to perform certain gestures on their own, while others require partial or total assistance. For example, a patient undergoing rehabilitation after orthopedic surgery may be able to wash his or her upper body on their own, but may need help to clean the lower parts of the body, notably due to restrictions of movement or pain. The caregiver must therefore adjust his or her assistance so as to enable the patient to participate in his or her own care as far as possible, while taking charge of the parts of care that the patient is unable to perform. This shared approach respects the patient's dignity, while encouraging him or her to maintain or regain a degree of autonomy.

When the patient is totally dependent, particularly in the event of paralysis, extreme weakness or after major surgery, the caregiver must **provide complete hygiene care**, taking care to limit painful or tiring movements for the patient. One of the techniques frequently used in these situations is bed hygiene. This must be carried out with great delicacy, taking care to protect vulnerable areas of the body, such as surgical areas, wounds or areas prone to bedsores. In these cases, the caregiver mobilizes the patient carefully, using gentle movements and supporting the parts of the body that need special protection. This passive mobilization both ensures complete hygiene and prevents the formation of prolonged pressure points, which can lead to skin complications.

In other situations, where the patient can be transferred but has significant **motor limitations**, such as muscular weakness or balance problems, toileting can be carried out in a **seated** position, on a shower chair or at the edge of the bed. Here, the caregiver adapts care according to the patient's stability and ability to participate. He or she must be vigilant with regard to the patient's posture, ensuring that he or she is correctly installed and secured, to avoid any risk of falling or becoming unbalanced. The use of adapted devices, such as non-slip shower seats or grab bars, is essential to guarantee the patient's safety throughout the care process. By adapting the toileting environment to the patient's physical condition, the caregiver helps to maintain an optimum level of comfort and safety, while respecting the patient's bodily integrity.

Adapting hygiene care to physical limitations also involves the **use of specific techniques**, such as part-washing. This method involves cleaning the patient's body step by step, uncovering only one part at a time, to limit exposure and maintain body heat. This technique is particularly useful for patients with respiratory or circulatory disorders, who may be sensitive to temperature variations. Similarly, for patients suffering from chronic pain or inflammation, the caregiver should take care to use gentle gestures, avoid excessive friction and favor the use of moist wipes or no-rinse cleansing solutions, when contact with water is uncomfortable or impossible.

One of the most challenging aspects of adapting hygiene care to physical limitations is **preventing skin complications**, particularly pressure sores. Patients who are bedridden or have very limited mobility are particularly vulnerable to pressure sores, which can develop rapidly in the absence of appropriate care. By adapting the frequency of hygiene care and regularly moisturizing the skin in at-risk areas (heels, sacrum, elbows), caregivers play a key role in preventing these lesions. In addition, during treatment, it is essential to regularly reposition the patient, ensuring that the parts of the body most exposed to pressure are well protected. The use of specific equipment, such as positioning cushions or anti-bedsore mattresses, is also central to adapting hygiene care to the needs of at-risk patients.

Finally, it is essential that the caregiver, while adapting care to physical limitations, remains **attentive to** the patient's **psychological aspect**. Personal hygiene, particularly when the patient is dependent, can be a moment of emotional vulnerability. Loss of autonomy, especially in such intimate gestures as grooming, can make some patients feel embarrassed or humiliated. It is therefore crucial that the caregiver also adapts his or her relational approach, demonstrating great sensitivity and respect. Explaining every gesture, involving the patient as much as possible, and respecting his or her privacy (for example, by covering body parts that are not being cleaned) helps preserve dignity and reduce the emotional discomfort associated with dependency.

- Prevention of pressure sores and other complications associated with immobility.

The prevention of pressure sores and other complications associated with immobility is a fundamental issue in the care of rehabilitation patients, especially those who are partially or totally bedridden. Prolonged immobility, often unavoidable in this context, entails major health risks, including the development of pressure sores, circulatory, respiratory and muscular disorders. The nursing auxiliary plays a crucial role in preventing these complications, by adopting a proactive approach and implementing adapted care aimed at protecting the patient from the harmful effects of immobility, while maintaining his or her comfort and well-being.

Pressure sores, also known as pressure ulcers, are skin lesions that develop when the skin and underlying tissues are compressed for long periods, resulting in poor blood circulation. The most vulnerable areas are those where the bones are close to the skin surface, such as the heels, sacrum, hips or elbows. The key to preventing pressure sores is constant monitoring and careful skin care. Caregivers must regularly inspect at-risk areas for the first signs of pressure sores, such as persistent redness, hardening of the skin or changes in texture. Early detection means early intervention, before pressure sores form and become a serious complication.

One of the first measures to prevent pressure sores is **regular repositioning of** the patient. A bedridden patient, unable to move independently, needs to be repositioned at least every two hours to relieve pressure on vulnerable areas. The caregiver, using appropriate mobilization techniques, ensures that the patient's position is gently changed, while making sure that the new positions are comfortable and safe. This change of position helps to restore blood flow to compressed areas and reduce the risk of injury. When repositioning, the caregiver must also ensure that the patient is not placed on folds of bed linen or other objects that could increase pressure on certain areas of the body.

The use of **technical aids** is also essential to prevent pressure sores. Devices such as anti-pressure sore mattresses, positioning cushions or foam cushions can reduce pressure on sensitive areas of the body. These devices distribute the patient's weight more evenly, minimizing pressure points. The caregiver must ensure that these devices are correctly installed and adapted to the patient's specific needs. For example, for a patient who is permanently bedridden, a dynamic air mattress, which alternates pressure points by inflating and deflating air cells, can be an effective solution for reducing the risk of pressure sores.

In addition to preventing bedsores, prolonged immobility also exposes patients to other complications, notably **respiratory disorders**. Bedridden patients are often less able to breathe deeply, which can lead to a build-up of secretions in the lungs, increasing the risk of respiratory infections such as pneumonia. The caregiver, in collaboration with the medical team, should encourage patients to perform regular breathing exercises, if their condition allows, to maintain good lung capacity. Techniques such as deep breathing or the use of an incentive spirometer can be implemented to help patients ventilate their lungs correctly. In cases where the patient is too weak to perform these exercises, interventions such as postural drainage or positioning aids can be used to facilitate the evacuation of secretions.

Immobility can also lead to **circulatory complications**, including the risk of blood clots, or deep vein thrombosis (DVT), which often develop in the legs as a result of blood stagnation in the veins. To prevent these thromboses, the caregiver must encourage **passive mobilization of the** lower limbs, by performing gentle mobilization exercises on the patient's legs and feet. Even if the patient is unable to move on his or her own, these passive movements, such as flexing and extending the feet, stimulate blood circulation and help prevent the formation of clots. In parallel, the use of compression stockings or intermittent compression devices may also be prescribed to promote blood circulation and reduce the risk of thrombosis.

Another risk associated with prolonged immobility is **muscle loss**, or sarcopenia, which can occur when muscles are not used. This muscle atrophy leads to a loss of strength and mobility, making the patient's recovery even more difficult. To prevent this complication, the caregiver should encourage **active mobilization** of the patient wherever possible. This may include simple exercises performed in bed, such as bending the arms or legs, or attempting to sit or stand with assistance. These exercises must be adapted to the patient's state of health and be progressive, to avoid excessive fatigue or injury. The caregiver, in collaboration with the physiotherapist, helps to maintain the patient's muscle mass and flexibility, even in situations of limited mobility.

Finally, a fundamental aspect of preventing immobility-related complications is **monitoring** the patient's **nutritional and hydration status.** Good nutrition is essential to preserve skin integrity and promote healing, while adequate hydration helps maintain skin elasticity and prevent urinary tract infections, which are often favored by immobility. The caregiver, by ensuring that the patient receives balanced meals and regular hydration, plays a key role in the overall support of the patient's health. They can also point out any difficulties with eating or drinking, which may require dietary adaptations, such as the introduction of protein-rich foods or thickened drinks for patients with swallowing disorders.

Assistance with mobilization and pain management
- Techniques to assist mobilization without aggravating lesions.

Assisting patient mobilization while avoiding aggravating existing lesions is a crucial aspect of the caregiver's work, particularly in rehabilitation. Patient mobilization, whether active or passive, plays a fundamental role in preventing complications associated with immobility, such as pressure sores, muscle contractures or thrombosis, while facilitating the restoration of mobility and autonomy. However, to be effective and safe, mobilization must be performed with care, taking into account the patient's physical limitations and any underlying pathologies, such as fractures, recent surgery or chronic pain. Mobilization techniques must therefore be adapted and precise, to encourage movement without aggravating lesions or causing new pain.

One of the first rules to follow is to **assess the patient's condition** before each mobilization attempt. The caregiver must take into account the patient's current physical condition: his or her ability to move independently, pain, any post-operative restrictions or injuries. For example, a patient who has undergone hip or knee surgery will not be mobilized in the same way as a stroke patient with partial paralysis. This assessment helps determine the best approach to mobilization, whether it's simply helping the patient to reposition in bed, or supporting them during a transfer from bed to chair.

Next, it's essential to **prepare the environment** and ensure that all the necessary equipment is at hand. If mobilization involves transferring the patient from bed to chair or wheelchair, the caregiver must check that the bed and wheelchair brakes are engaged to prevent sudden movement. Ensuring that the floor is clear and free of obstacles, and using technical aids such as support bars, positioning cushions or sliding sheets will also facilitate mobilization and reduce the risk of injury. Adequate preparation of the space and suitable devices ensure the safety of both patient and caregiver, while making mobilization smoother and more comfortable.

Transfer techniques are essential to help mobilize patients while protecting vulnerable areas. For example, for a bedridden patient who needs to be repositioned or straightened in bed, the use of the **rolling** technique is particularly effective. This technique involves gently rolling the patient onto his or her side, supporting the body so as to minimize strain on sensitive joints or pressure points. Rolling also reduces friction and the risk of skin shearing, which can lead to pressure sores. By using a sliding sheet or transfer sheet, the caregiver can mobilize the patient more easily and gently, while avoiding pulling directly on the patient's body, which could aggravate injury or pain.

When the patient has to be **seated or transferred out of bed**, it is crucial to adopt a progressive mobilization technique to avoid causing vertigo or imbalance. When transferring from a bed to a chair, the caregiver begins by helping the patient to sit on the edge of the bed, supporting his or her back and placing the patient's feet firmly on the floor. This sitting position enables the patient to regain his or her bearings before getting up. Then, by maintaining stable physical contact, the caregiver can accompany the patient in the transition from sitting to standing. If the patient is able to stand unaided but needs support, the caregiver can use a **transfer belt**, placed around the patient's waist, to provide additional support while maintaining control over the movement. This technique enables the patient to actively participate in the transfer, while avoiding stressing injured or weakened areas.

During **passive mobilizations**, which involve patients who are unable to move on their own, it is essential to perform movements with great gentleness, while maintaining adequate support for the limbs. For example, when mobilizing an upper or lower limb, the caregiver supports the limb so as to spread the load over the entire area to be mobilized, taking care not to pull directly on joints or muscles. Slow, fluid movements, such as flexing and extending the arms or legs, help maintain joint flexibility without causing pain or aggravating an existing injury. These passive mobilizations help prevent muscle contractures and maintain adequate blood circulation, while avoiding the onset of joint stiffness.

In some cases, such as for patients with fractures or who have undergone surgery, the caregiver must ensure that **specific medical instructions are followed**. For example, after hip surgery, the patient must not bend the hip more than 90 degrees, nor cross the legs. Caregivers must therefore be vigilant in respecting these limitations during transfers or mobilizations, to avoid any risk of dislocation or post-operative complications. By carefully following doctors' and physiotherapists' instructions, the caregiver helps to protect the patient, while facilitating faster recovery.

Dialogue with the patient is also an essential component of mobilization. Even in the case of very weak patients or those with communication difficulties, it's important to always explain the movements you're going to perform, and to invite the patient to participate as much as possible. This reassures the patient and encourages him or her to take an active part in rehabilitation, while reducing anxiety. The caregiver can also solicit feedback from the patient regarding pain or discomfort during mobilization, so as to adjust the movements or technique used according to the patient's sensations.

Finally, it is essential that the caregiver **adopts correct posture** when mobilizing the patient, to avoid injuring himself or herself. Carrying techniques based on good ergonomics, such as bending the knees rather than the back, using leg strength to lift, or keeping the back straight and feet firmly planted on the floor, help protect the caregiver while ensuring safe and efficient patient mobilization. The use of technical aids, such as patient lifts or transfer boards, is also recommended where necessary, to minimize physical effort and ensure safe transfer.

- Pain monitoring and collaboration with the team for relief.

Monitoring pain in rehabilitation patients is an essential task in ensuring their comfort and optimizing their recovery. Pain, whether acute or chronic, is a factor that can not only slow down the rehabilitation process, but also have a negative impact on patient morale, reducing their motivation to participate actively in care. By being in direct and constant contact with patients, caregivers play a key role in detecting, assessing and communicating the pain they feel. This careful monitoring enables them to collaborate effectively with the care team to adjust treatments and implement appropriate strategies to relieve pain.

The first aspect of pain monitoring is **regular assessment of** its intensity and nature. Pain can fluctuate over the course of a day, and its causes can vary according to movements, the care provided or the patient's underlying pathologies. Caregivers often use specific tools, such as the **Visual Analog Scale (VAS)**, which enables patients to quantify their pain on a scale of 1 to 10. This simple and effective method provides precise data on pain, not only in terms of intensity, but also in terms of its evolution over time. By asking open-ended questions about the location, duration and nature of the pain (for example, whether it is stabbing, acute, or diffuse), the caregiver can gather detailed information that will facilitate the adjustment of care.

At the same time, some patients, especially those with communication disorders, cognitive deficits or difficulties expressing their feelings, may find it difficult to verbalize their pain. In such cases, the caregiver must **watch for non-verbal signs** of pain, such as grimaces, changes in posture, agitation, facial expressions of suffering or moaning. These often subtle signs can reveal pain that is not expressed verbally. Through careful observation, the caregiver is able to detect these manifestations and alert the medical team. They can also observe the impact of pain on daily activities, such as reluctance to move, difficulty walking or getting up, which may indicate physical suffering.

Once pain has been identified and assessed, it is crucial to **communicate quickly and effectively** with the care team to adjust management. Here, the caregiver acts as a relay between the patient and the rest of the team, passing on information gathered during care and reporting any significant changes in the intensity or location of the pain. This communication can take place during oral or written transmissions, where the caregiver details his or her observations and reports pain assessment data. The nursing team, made up of nurses, doctors and physiotherapists, can then react by adjusting drug treatments, modifying the rehabilitation program or proposing alternative pain relief solutions.

In many cases, pain relief involves **therapeutic adjustments**, such as modifying doses of analgesics, anti-inflammatories or opioids, under the supervision of the physician. The caregiver, in collaboration with the nurses, carefully monitors the effectiveness of these treatments. He or she assesses whether pain is relieved after the medication has been administered, whether there are any side effects, and whether any adjustments need to be made. The evolution of pain after drug treatment is a key indicator for the medical team, who can, if necessary, re-evaluate the treatment strategy to offer optimal relief.

In addition to drug treatments, the caregiver can help implement **non-pharmacological methods** to relieve pain. These complementary techniques, often used alongside drug treatments, include measures such as the application of heat or cold to painful areas, relaxation techniques, or light massage. For example, a warm compress can be applied to relax stiff muscles, while a cold compress can help reduce inflammation after rehabilitation exercise. These interventions, although seemingly simple, can bring significant relief and are particularly suitable for muscle or joint pain.

Another important aspect of pain management is **adapting care** to avoid exacerbating existing pain. By being attentive to the patient's reactions, the caregiver must adapt his or her actions according to the pain reported. For example, during hygiene care or transfers, it is essential to avoid sudden movements that could intensify pain, especially in the case of patients with fractures, surgery or osteoarthritis. By correctly supporting painful body parts and using gentle, progressive techniques to mobilize the patient, the caregiver minimizes the risk of pain worsening.

Finally, the caregiver's role is not limited to assessment and transmission of information; it also includes important **psychological support.** Pain, especially chronic pain, can provoke anxiety, frustration and feelings of helplessness in patients. The caregiver's reassuring presence, attentiveness and empathy can help the patient to manage his or her pain more effectively. They can encourage them to verbalize their feelings, express their fears or ask questions about current treatments. By establishing a relationship of trust, the caregiver helps the patient to feel cared for and listened to, which helps to reduce pain-related anxiety and, in some cases, to improve the perception of pain itself.

Nutrition and hydration for rehabilitation patients
- Adapt meals to the patient's condition: assistance, monitoring of specific diets.

Adapting meals to the patient's condition is an essential step in ensuring good nutrition, preventing complications and supporting the rehabilitation process. Each rehabilitation patient has specific needs, depending on his or her physical condition, pathologies, ability to feed himself or herself, and the diets prescribed by doctors. The caregiver plays a key role in assisting with meals and monitoring specific diets, to ensure that patients receive a diet adapted to their needs while respecting their limitations.

Mealtime assistance can take different forms, depending on the patient's level of autonomy. Some patients, although able to feed themselves, may require adjustments to facilitate their meal. For example, patients with motor or coordination problems, such as those who have suffered a stroke, may have difficulty using cutlery or maintaining a firm grip on utensils. In such cases, the caregiver can suggest **technical aids**, such as adapted cutlery with wider handles or spouted cups, which facilitate gripping and enable the patient to eat alone as much as possible. This approach helps preserve the patient's autonomy, while making eating more comfortable and less frustrating.

For patients who are unable to feed themselves because of their physical limitations, the caregiver must provide **full assistance** during the meal. This involves feeding the patient in a slow, measured manner, while remaining attentive to the patient's rhythm and reactions. It is important to respect the patient's comfort by adopting a comfortable sitting position, with adequate back and arm support, and to ensure that the food is at the right temperature to avoid the risk of burns or discomfort. The caregiver must also be attentive to the texture of food, ensuring that it is adapted to the patient's chewing and swallowing abilities. For example, for patients with swallowing difficulties (dysphagia), it may be necessary to modify the texture of food by grinding or thickening it to facilitate ingestion and avoid the risk of choking.

Monitoring specific diets is another crucial aspect of meal adaptation. Many rehabilitation patients have to follow special diets depending on their pathology, such as salt-free diets for patients suffering from hypertension, diabetic diets for those who need to control their blood sugar levels, or protein-rich diets to promote muscle recovery after surgery. Caregivers must ensure that the meals they serve scrupulously comply with the dietary instructions prescribed by doctors and dieticians. This includes checking meal trays to ensure that food corresponds to the patient's diet and, if necessary, pointing out any inconsistencies so that adjustments can be made.

It's also important to take into account any **food allergies** or intolerances the patient may have. Certain allergies, such as those to gluten, dairy products or seafood, can lead to serious complications if not respected. Caregivers must be vigilant to ensure that patients do not come into contact with forbidden foods, even accidentally. This careful monitoring helps prevent allergic reactions and ensures that the patient's diet is not only nutritious, but also safe.

In addition to specific diets, the caregiver must pay particular attention to **the quantity and frequency of meals**, especially for patients who may have difficulty maintaining a good nutritional status. Some patients, because of their state of health or treatment, may lose their appetite, suffer from nausea or have difficulty finishing their meals. In such cases, the caregiver must ensure that these patients are given suitable portions, and encouraged to eat small quantities more frequently, if necessary. It is also essential to monitor food intake to identify any weight loss or signs of malnutrition, and report these observations to the medical team to adjust the meal plan accordingly.

Hydration is another often overlooked but equally important aspect of meal management. Bedridden or rehabilitated patients may not feel thirsty, which increases the risk of dehydration, especially in the elderly or those on diuretic therapy. Caregivers must ensure that patients drink regularly, adapting the quantities and frequency of water intake to their condition. For patients with swallowing difficulties, it may be necessary to thicken liquids to make them easier to swallow, without risking false routes. Hydration is a key factor in maintaining physiological equilibrium, and helps support bodily functions essential to healing.

The caregiver's role is not limited to supervision and assistance. It's also important to **involve the patient in their meal** as much as possible, giving them choices, even when on a special diet. Asking the patient if he prefers one food to another, or if he wishes to eat at a particular time, reinforces his sense of autonomy and control over his daily life, which is essential for his psychological well-being. Meals can thus become moments of comfort and pleasure, rather than a simple functional necessity.

Finally, the caregiver must **communicate regularly with the medical team and dieticians** to report any difficulties related to the patient's nutrition. If a patient refuses to eat, shows signs of malnutrition or intolerance, or expresses pain or discomfort during meals, this information must be passed on to the care team in order to adjust the nutritional plan. Changes in the patient's state of health, whether related to pathology or rehabilitation, may require modifications to the diet, and the caregiver is often best placed to spot these early signs.

- Promote independent eating while maintaining safety.

Promoting autonomy in eating, while maintaining safety, is a delicate but essential balance to achieve in order to support rehabilitation and boost patients' self-confidence. In rehabilitation, meals represent much more than a simple nutritional need: they are a key stage in the regaining of autonomy, a moment when the patient can gradually regain functional independence. However, depending on the patient's state of health, this autonomy must be encouraged with care, taking particular care to ensure safety, especially in the event of motor, cognitive or swallowing difficulties. The caregiver plays a central role in this process, offering support tailored to each patient's individual needs, while helping them to master the gestures involved in eating.

The first step in promoting independent eating is to **create a suitable, safe environment**. This starts with putting the patient in a comfortable, stable position, usually seated, with feet firmly planted on the floor or supported, and back properly supported. If the patient is bedridden, it is essential to straighten the bed to an angle that facilitates swallowing, while guaranteeing sufficient support to avoid any imbalance. The caregiver must ensure that the table or meal tray is at the right height and within easy reach, so that the patient can reach his or her food without undue effort. The aim is to make every gesture accessible and easy, avoiding sudden or dangerous movements.

For some patients, especially those with **motor** or coordination **disorders** such as Parkinson's, stroke or tremors, specific **technical aids** can make meal-taking much easier. These can include ergonomic cutlery, designed with thicker or non-slip handles to make it easier to grip, or cups with spouts to prevent spills. Plates with sloping edges or non-slip plates can also help contain food and simplify handling. These devices enable patients to feed themselves, while reducing the risk of frustration or accidents, such as dropping utensils or spilling food.

The caregiver should also encourage the patient's **active participation** in mealtimes. Even if the patient requires partial assistance, it is important to let him/her perform the gestures that he/she is capable of doing alone, offering discreet support when necessary. For example, a patient may be able to bring a spoon to his or her mouth, but need help cutting food. The caregiver can then intervene for this task, while allowing the patient to continue eating independently. This approach boosts the patient's self-confidence and encourages him or her to continue striving towards more complete autonomy, while maintaining safe supervision.

Vigilance with regard to swallowing is paramount, especially for patients with swallowing disorders (dysphagia), who may be at risk of false routes, choking or food inhalation. In these cases, the caregiver must adapt the consistency of the food to make it easier to swallow. For example, food can be blended or thickened to prevent it going down the throat too quickly. The patient should be encouraged to eat slowly, taking small bites and chewing well before swallowing. The caregiver can remain close by to monitor safety throughout the meal, intervening quickly if necessary, but without interfering excessively with the patient's initiative.

In some cases, it can be helpful to set up **routines** that help patients structure their meals. This can include presenting food in an organized way, explaining what types of food are on the tray and how they are arranged, particularly for patients with cognitive or memory impairments. By guiding the patient through the steps of the meal, the caregiver fosters a sense of control and understanding, while maintaining a reassuring and secure environment. This approach is particularly beneficial for patients suffering from dementia or Alzheimer's, who may have difficulty finding their bearings in space or remembering what to do.

The caregiver must also be **attentive to** the patient's **fatigue**. Eating can represent a considerable effort for some people undergoing rehabilitation, and it is important to adapt the pace of the meal to their energy levels. If a patient shows signs of exhaustion or discouragement, it's essential to give them time to rest before resuming. The aim is not to rush the meal, to preserve the pleasure of eating and prevent the patient from feeling overwhelmed by the task.

Throughout this process, the caregiver must **acknowledge the** patient's progress, however modest it may seem. Every gesture made independently, every mouthful taken without help, is a step towards autonomy. Encouraging and congratulating the patient on his or her efforts helps to boost motivation and self-esteem. It is essential to understand that rehabilitation is not limited to physiotherapy or functional rehabilitation exercises: every meal is an opportunity for the patient to regain possession of his or her body and movements, in a concrete, everyday setting.

Finally, **regular observations of** the patient at mealtimes should be shared with the rest of the care team. If a patient progresses and manages to perform certain gestures alone, it may be necessary to readjust the level of assistance at subsequent meals. Conversely, if the patient shows increasing difficulties or new complications, such as swallowing problems or loss of strength, this information should be passed on to the team to consider modifications to the care plan or dietary adaptations.

Chapter 4

Actively participate in the rehabilitation process

Collaboration with physiotherapists and occupational therapists

○ Help in preparing rehabilitation sessions.

Helping patients prepare for rehabilitation sessions is a key task, ensuring that they approach these moments in optimal conditions, both physically and psychologically. In rehabilitation, each rehabilitation session represents a step towards recovery and regaining autonomy. However, for these sessions to be effective and safe, it is essential that the patient is well prepared. The caregiver plays a central role in this preparation, ensuring that the patient is physically ready, motivated and in a mental state conducive to rehabilitation, while collaborating with the team of physiotherapists, occupational therapists and other health professionals to optimize the sessions.

The first step in preparing a patient for a rehabilitation session is to **ensure their physical comfort**. It is essential to check that the patient is suitably settled before starting the session. If the patient is bedridden or has difficulty moving, the caregiver ensures that the transfer to the rehabilitation room is safe. This may involve the use of a wheelchair, walker or other mobility aids. The patient's set-up must be comfortable, but also practical, to enable good participation in the exercises. For example, for a physiotherapy session focusing on leg mobility, it is important that the patient is seated correctly, with feet firmly planted on the floor and legs in a position that allows the exercises to be performed without discomfort.

The caregiver also **checks the** patient's **general physical condition** before the session. This involves ensuring that the patient is sufficiently rested, and has no excessive pain or signs of unusual fatigue. If the patient reports intense pain or discomfort, it is crucial to take this into account, as it could compromise the quality of rehabilitation or aggravate an existing condition. In this case, the caregiver can adjust the level of support or inform the rehabilitation team so that the session is adapted to the patient's condition. Sometimes, this may involve minor adjustments, such as reducing the intensity of exercises or lengthening the rest periods between each effort.

Equally important is the patient's **psychological preparation**. Rehabilitation sessions can be demanding, both physically and mentally, especially for patients facing significant limitations or slow progress. The caregiver plays a moral support role, ensuring that the patient is ready to commit fully to the session. This can include encouragement, explanations of the session's objectives, or reassuring words to allay fears or frustrations. It's important that the patient understands the meaning and importance of the exercises he or she is about to perform, as this reinforces motivation and involvement. By establishing an open and empathetic dialogue, the caregiver helps the patient to approach the session with greater serenity and confidence in his or her abilities.

In addition to emotional support, the caregiver can **prepare the necessary equipment** for the rehabilitation session. Each type of exercise requires specific equipment, whether elastic bands, rehabilitation balls, parallel bars or exercise machines. The caregiver, in collaboration with the rehabilitation team, ensures that all equipment is available, in good condition and ready for use. For example, for a lower limb rehabilitation session, the caregiver may ensure that the support bars are properly positioned, that mobilization accessories are ready, or that safety devices such as support belts are available if required. This material preparation allows the session to begin without delay, while ensuring that each exercise is carried out under optimum conditions.

When preparing a session, it is also essential to **take into account** the patient's **specific needs**. Each patient has different goals and abilities, and the caregiver must ensure that the session is adapted to these particularities. For example, if a patient needs special support to move to the rehabilitation room, or if accommodations need to be made because of recent pain or a temporary limitation, the caregiver ensures that everything is in place to facilitate the session. This careful monitoring enables us to personalize the treatment and adapt the exercises to the patient's abilities and needs, without compromising comfort or safety.

At the same time, the caregiver may be involved in **managing medical parameters** before and after the session. Blood pressure, heart rate and oxygen saturation are often measured prior to the session, particularly for patients with cardiac or respiratory problems. These data enable the rehabilitation team to adapt the exercises to the patient's state of health at that particular moment. The caregiver plays a crucial role in this monitoring, transmitting the necessary information to the multidisciplinary team. Likewise, after the session, he or she may need to check these parameters to ensure that the patient has recovered well and has not developed complications linked to the effort.

Managing the post-session is just as important as preparing for it. Once rehabilitation is complete, the caregiver ensures that the patient is comfortably reinstalled, rested and hydrated. He or she is also attentive to the patient's emotional state after the effort: if the patient appears discouraged or tired, the caregiver can play a supportive role by acknowledging the progress made, however small. This recognition of effort is vital to maintain the patient's commitment to the long rehabilitation process.

- Effort monitoring and support for rehabilitation activities.

Effort monitoring and support during rehabilitation activities are essential aspects in ensuring that each session is both safe and beneficial for the patient. Rehabilitation exercises are often demanding, both physically and mentally, and it's crucial to strike the right balance between asking enough of the patient to encourage progress, without overtaxing them or worsening their condition. The caregiver, working closely with rehabilitation professionals, plays a key role in this dynamic. They ensure that the patient respects his or her limits, while encouraging them to gently push back their abilities, all within a secure framework.

Effort monitoring begins with careful observation of the patient's reactions during exercise. Every patient reacts differently to exertion, and it is essential to be alert to signs of fatigue, pain or shortness of breath. The caregiver must be able to recognize these signs early, by observing such things as accelerated breathing, changes in posture, grimaces or expressions of suffering, as well as verbalized complaints of pain. This vigilance makes it possible to interrupt or adapt exercise immediately if necessary, to prevent any risk of injury or overexertion. For example, if a patient shows signs of muscle weakness or exhaustion during a walking exercise, it may be necessary to take a break, reduce the intensity of the exercise, or offer more active support.

In addition to visible signs of fatigue, the caregiver can use assessment tools such as the **Borg scale**, which measures the patient's perception of effort. By asking the patient to rate the intensity of exercise on a scale of 1 to 10, it is possible to adapt exercises in real time, ensuring that effort remains within a tolerable and productive zone for the patient. This monitoring helps to avoid situations where the patient might exceed his or her limits without being fully aware of it. This subjective assessment, combined with clinical observation, ensures that rehabilitation activities are carried out safely.

Physical support during rehabilitation sessions is also a crucial part of the caregiver's job. Exercises, whether involving mobility, muscle strength or balance, may require active assistance from the caregiver to ensure the patient's safety. For example, during walking exercises, the caregiver may use a **transfer belt** to support the patient and help maintain balance, while remaining ready to intervene in the event of an imbalance or fall. This type of support enables the patient to concentrate on the exercise, knowing that he or she is safe, thus boosting confidence and motivation to progress.

Technical aids such as walkers, walking sticks or parallel bars may also be required for walking and transfer rehabilitation. The caregiver ensures that these devices are properly adjusted and adapted to the patient's physical capabilities. They help patients to use these aids correctly and safely, accompanying them in their movements and ensuring that each gesture is carried out smoothly and without risk. This support is particularly important for patients who are gradually regaining their mobility, but who are not yet stable enough to move around without assistance.

In addition to the physical aspect, the caregiver provides crucial **moral support** throughout the rehabilitation sessions. Rehabilitation can be a long and difficult process, where progress is not always immediately visible. Some patients may become discouraged, frustrated or lose confidence in their abilities. The caregiver's constant listening and encouragement help maintain a positive frame of mind. He or she rewards every bit of progress, however small, and reminds the patient of the importance of persevering. This moral support, often discreet but fundamental, helps to reinforce the patient's motivation and enable him or her to continue their efforts with greater zest.

It is also important to respect **recovery times** during and after exercises. The caregiver ensures that the patient is not pushed beyond his or her limits, and allows regular breaks to avoid exhaustion. These moments of rest are also an opportunity to assess the patient's general condition, check vitals (such as pulse and respiration), and ensure that he or she is ready to continue exercising or that it is time to stop the session. Recovery is a crucial stage in maximizing the benefits of exercise, while avoiding the risk of overexertion or complications.

After each rehabilitation session, the caregiver plays an important role in **calming the patient down** and providing post-exercise follow-up. This includes making the patient comfortable again, ensuring they are well hydrated and rested, and checking for any new or unusual pain. If the patient reports persistent pain or discomfort after the session, the caregiver can adjust care or alert the medical team to re-evaluate the exercises prescribed. This post-exercise monitoring enables us to anticipate possible complications and adjust future sessions to the patient's condition.

Lastly, **communication with the multidisciplinary team** is essential for adjusting rehabilitation sessions in line with observations made during exercises. Nurses pass on their comments to physiotherapists, occupational therapists and other health professionals, indicating progress made, difficulties encountered or adjustments required. For example, if a patient shows signs of progress in muscle strength, the team may decide to gradually increase the intensity of exercises. Conversely, if the patient is experiencing increasing difficulties, an adaptation of the rehabilitation program may be considered to better suit his or her current abilities.

Encouraging and motivating patients on a daily basis

- Strategies to boost patient motivation.

Reinforcing the motivation of rehabilitation patients is an essential component of their care. Rehabilitation, which is often long and sometimes frustrating, can test patients' patience and determination, especially when progress is slow or physical limitations persist. In this context, the caregiver plays a key role in stimulating and maintaining patient motivation, using a variety of strategies that combine psychological support, progressive encouragement and the creation of an environment conducive to rehabilitation. These strategies not only improve adherence to care, but also give patients the energy they need to actively engage in their recovery journey.

One of the first strategies for boosting patient motivation is to **set realistic, achievable goals**. When goals are too ambitious or ill-defined, patients can quickly feel discouraged, especially if they feel they are not making progress. The caregiver, in collaboration with the multidisciplinary team, can help break down the rehabilitation journey into smaller, achievable steps. For example, rather than focusing on the ultimate goal of walking unassisted, it is more motivating for a patient to aim first for the ability to stand up unaided, or to walk a few metres with a technical aid. By achieving these small intermediate goals, patients can see their progress, which boosts their confidence and their desire to continue.

Another important motivating factor **is constant encouragement**. The caregiver, through his or her daily presence and support, can play a crucial role in valuing every effort made by the patient. It's important to congratulate successes, even the most modest ones, and to recognize progress, even when it's not spectacular. For example, a patient who manages to achieve a more fluid movement or transfer with less difficulty deserves encouragement. This reinforces the patient's sense of pride and encourages him or her to keep up the good work. The caregiver can also remind the patient of progress made over a longer period, to show that, despite moments of stagnation or difficulty, significant advances have been made since the beginning of the rehabilitation process.

Psychological support is also essential to maintain motivation. Rehabilitation can be challenging not only physically, but also mentally. Some patients may be tempted to give up, or become overwhelmed by frustration at their limitations. The caregiver, by listening and empathizing, can help soothe these feelings of discouragement by providing a space where the patient can express his or her fears and frustrations. By responding sympathetically to these concerns and reassuring the patient of his or her ability to overcome difficulties, the caregiver helps to restore the patient's self-confidence. This moral support is particularly crucial at times when the patient doubts his or her ability to recover, or feels discouraged by slow progress.

A complementary strategy is to **personalize rehabilitation sessions** to make them more engaging and tailored to the patient's interests. By knowing the patient well, the caregiver can suggest activities that correspond to his or her tastes, or that recall everyday gestures. For example, for a patient who enjoyed gardening before hospitalization, exercises that imitate the movements involved in this activity (bending over, lifting objects) can make rehabilitation more meaningful and motivating. By incorporating familiar or pleasurable elements, the caregiver makes the exercises less daunting and anchors them in the prospect of a return to an active life.

What's more, it's important to **involve the patient in the decision-making process**. Motivation is often heightened when patients feel in control of their own choices, and involved in their own recovery. The caregiver can encourage the patient to participate in the design of his or her rehabilitation program by asking for his or her opinion on certain aspects: does he or she prefer to do one exercise before another? Would he like to adapt the pace of the session? By giving the patient some leeway, the caregiver helps to reinforce his or her commitment to, and responsibility for, his or her own rehabilitation process. This partial autonomy gives the patient a sense of control, which can boost his or her motivation to achieve set goals.

Adapting sessions to the day's capabilities is also an important strategy for avoiding discouragement. Every day is different for a rehabilitation patient: some days, they may feel more energetic and capable of great effort, while on other days, they may be more tired or in greater pain. The caregiver must be able to recognize these variations and adjust the exercises accordingly. By modifying the intensity or duration of exercises according to the patient's condition, the caregiver enables the patient to progress at his or her own pace, without the risk of pushing him or her too far, which could lead to exhaustion or frustration.

Encouragement to set personal goals can also boost motivation. Beyond the rehabilitation goals prescribed by the medical team, patients can set goals that are important to them, such as regaining autonomy to perform a specific task, like cooking, dressing themselves, or even resuming an activity they used to enjoy. By helping the patient to achieve these personal goals, the caregiver gives him or her an additional reason to commit fully to the rehabilitation process, as these objectives have a direct bearing on quality of life.

Finally, the **involvement of family and friends** can be a valuable source of motivation. Family support plays a key role in patient recovery. The caregiver can encourage the family to take part in rehabilitation sessions, or to support the patient in his or her efforts. Seeing the progress made in the eyes of loved ones, or knowing that recovery will facilitate a return to family life, can motivate the patient to pursue his or her efforts with greater determination. By creating a supportive environment where the patient feels surrounded and encouraged, the caregiver helps to reinforce his or her commitment.

- Dealing with frustrations and psychological blockages.

Dealing with frustrations and psychological blockages is a fundamental aspect of supporting rehabilitation patients. The road to recovery is often strewn with physical and emotional challenges, which can slow progress or even discourage patients altogether. Frustrations frequently arise from the perception that progress is slow, that lost abilities are slow to return, or that set goals seem unattainable. These psychological blockages can become a real obstacle to rehabilitation if they are not taken into account. By being close to the patient, the caregiver plays a central role in identifying and managing these moments of discouragement. With an empathetic approach and appropriate strategies, they can help patients overcome their frustrations and regain the motivation they need to continue their efforts.

One of the first steps in dealing with frustration is to **actively listen to the patient**. Many patients feel a deep sense of injustice or powerlessness in the face of their physical limitations, and it is essential to offer them a space where they can freely express their emotions. The caregiver must be able to take in these frustrations in a non-judgmental, caring way. Sometimes, the simple fact of having someone to talk to, of being able to put their feelings into words, can help the patient evacuate some of the emotional charge that is preventing them from moving forward. This attentive listening also enables the caregiver to better understand the sources of frustration, whether it's a goal deemed too ambitious, pain that's poorly managed, or a feeling of loneliness in the face of hardship.

After listening to the patient, it's important to **help him reformulate his expectations**. Rehabilitation is often perceived as a long and uncertain process, where progress may seem invisible on a day-to-day basis. The caregiver can help reframe this perception by reminding the patient that every little improvement counts, even if it doesn't seem spectacular. By breaking down goals into smaller, achievable steps, it becomes easier for the patient to see concrete progress. For example, if a patient is frustrated at not yet being able to walk unaided, the caregiver can show them that the simple fact of walking longer or with less pain than before is already an encouraging sign. This helps restore the patient's confidence in his or her abilities, and reduces the sense of stagnation that fuels frustration.

Another crucial aspect of managing psychological blocks is **recognizing and validating the patient's emotions**. When patients feel understood in their suffering, they are more inclined to overcome their blocks. The caregiver can express empathy by recognizing that the difficulties encountered are real and legitimate. For example, he or she can tell the patient that it's normal to feel frustrated by the constant effort required in rehabilitation, or that it's understandable to feel discouraged by slow progress. This validation of emotions helps patients feel less alone in their experience, and helps them accept their frustrations rather than fight or deny them.

Encouraging patience and perseverance is another essential strategy for overcoming blockages. By showing constant support, the caregiver helps the patient understand that recovery takes time, and that perseverance is the key to success. It's important to remember that rehabilitation is a gradual process, and that even small victories accumulated day after day eventually lead to significant improvements. For example, the caregiver can remind the patient that there are ups and downs in every rehabilitation journey, and that a more difficult day does not mean that all efforts have been in vain. This long-term vision helps to reduce the pressure of day-to-day life and maintain motivation, even when progress is less obvious.

Suggesting alternatives or adaptations to rehabilitation exercises is also an effective way of getting around blockages. Some patients may be frustrated by the repetitiveness of exercises, or by the difficulty of certain movements. In such cases, the caregiver, in collaboration with the physiotherapist, can suggest variations that better match the patient's current abilities, or that add a more playful aspect to the sessions. For example, if a muscle-strengthening exercise is too painful or discouraging, it can be replaced by an activity that calls on the same muscle groups, but in a more motivating context, such as a game or a simulation of an everyday task. This allows the patient to rediscover the pleasure of effort and feel capable again.

Another effective strategy is to **value long-term progress**. It's easy for a patient to focus on what they can't yet do, but the caregiver can get them to look back and recognize how much they've already accomplished. By tracing the progress made since the start of rehabilitation, whether in terms of mobility, strength or pain management, the patient can better perceive how far he or she has come. The caregiver can also suggest that the patient keeps a rehabilitation diary, in which he or she notes daily progress, however small. This helps the patient to keep a visible record of his or her progress and become aware of successes, which can considerably reduce feelings of blockage.

Finally, the **management of psychological blockages** must include support tailored to the particularities of each patient. Some patients will need a softer, more reassuring approach, while others will respond better to more dynamic encouragement. It's important for the caregiver to adapt his or her speech and approach to each patient's temperament and emotional needs. In some cases, more structured support may be required, such as the intervention of a psychologist, to help the patient deal with feelings of depression or anxiety that can aggravate psychological blockages.

Psychosocial rehabilitation

- The caregiver's role in psychological support.

The caregiver's role in providing psychological support to patients is fundamental, especially in a rehabilitation setting, where the challenges are not only physical but also emotional. The rehabilitation process is often long and arduous, and patients find themselves confronted with new limitations, persistent pain and uncertainty about their recovery. In this context, the caregiver, by virtue of his or her daily proximity to the patient, becomes a privileged interlocutor to provide emotional support. They act not only as technical and medical support, but also as a resource person capable of listening, reassuring and motivating.

One of the first aspects of the caregiver's psychological support is **active listening**. In a medical context where patients can sometimes feel lost or isolated, it is essential for them to have someone to talk to about their fears, frustrations and hopes. The caregiver, through his or her constant presence, becomes this attentive ear, able to receive emotions without judgment. When a patient expresses his fear of not regaining his autonomy, or his frustration at his slow progress, the caregiver must be able to offer him a safe space in which to talk. This active listening not only recognizes the patient's psychological suffering, but also helps them to overcome it by verbalizing their concerns.

Reassurance is also an integral part of psychological support. Many patients undergoing rehabilitation can feel anxious, even distressed, when faced with the uncertainty of their physical future. Here, the caregiver plays a comforting role, providing reassuring answers and reminding the patient that he or she is surrounded by a competent, caring medical team. For example, when the patient worries that he or she is not progressing fast enough, the caregiver can remind him or her that each re-education session follows its own rhythm, and that even small steps forward are significant. This kind of soothing discourse helps to alleviate the patient's anxiety and give him or her a sense of security, essential for maintaining motivation.

Valuing progress is another way in which the caregiver can provide psychological support. The rehabilitation process is often punctuated by small victories, but also by moments of stagnation or apparent regression. It's easy for patients to focus on what they can't yet do, rather than on what they've already achieved. The caregiver has a key role to play in reminding the patient of his or her successes, however modest. For example, if a patient manages to walk a few steps further than the day before, or performs a gesture he or she was unable to do before, it is essential that the caregiver emphasizes this progress. This appreciation helps the patient to regain self-confidence and persevere in his or her efforts, despite the difficulties.

At the same time, the caregiver must demonstrate **constant empathy**, putting himself in the patient's shoes to better understand what he is going through. This empathetic attitude enables the patient to feel understood and supported, not only in his or her physical efforts, but also in his or her emotions. Empathy is expressed not only through words, but also through gestures: a reassuring smile, a hand on the shoulder, a shared moment of silence. These gestures, though they may seem insignificant, reinforce the relationship of trust between patient and caregiver, and help to create an environment where the patient feels emotionally secure.

Another essential aspect of psychological support is **adapting speech** and attitudes to the patient's personality and emotional needs. Some patients will need firm, regular encouragement to overcome their fears and physical limitations, while others will respond better to a softer, more reassuring approach. The caregiver, by knowing the patient well, needs to tailor his or her support to be as effective as possible. This involves understanding when the patient needs to be pushed to make an extra effort, and when they simply need to be listened to or reassured. This ability to adapt is essential to providing truly personalized and effective psychological support.

Support in dealing with frustrations and blockages is also an important part of the caregiver's role. In rehabilitation, patients are often confronted with moments of discouragement, when progress is less visible or even non-existent. These periods of stagnation can generate a great deal of frustration, leading to a psychological block. The caregiver's constant presence can help the patient overcome these moments by encouraging him or her not to give up, and by showing that these phases are an integral part of the rehabilitation process. They can also suggest adjustments to exercises or routines to make rehabilitation more dynamic and motivating. By helping the patient to overcome these blockages, the caregiver promotes not only physical progress, but also the patient's mental well-being.

Finally, the caregiver plays an important role in **preventing social isolation**. Rehabilitation patients, especially those who spend long periods in hospital or have lost some of their autonomy, can feel isolated or disconnected from their daily lives and loved ones. The caregiver, by encouraging social interaction, whether by facilitating family visits or encouraging patients to take part in group activities, helps to break down this isolation. Feeling surrounded and supported, both by the care team and by loved ones, boosts morale and gives patients the motivation they need to keep fighting.

- Help rebuild self-esteem and independence.

Helping to rebuild self-esteem and independence is an essential mission for caregivers in the patient rehabilitation process. After an accident, illness or surgery, many patients are faced with a loss of autonomy, sometimes sudden, which can profoundly affect their self-confidence. This loss of independence, whether temporary or permanent, often leads to feelings of frustration, inadequacy and vulnerability. In this context, the caregiver plays a fundamental role in helping patients gradually regain their dignity, self-esteem and ability to manage their daily lives. Through simple but essential gestures and constant psychological support, the caregiver helps to restore this self-confidence, step by step.

One of the first steps in rebuilding self-esteem is **to restore the patient's autonomy in everyday tasks**. Dependence on basic tasks, such as dressing, washing or feeding, can be a source of devaluation for the patient. The caregiver must therefore encourage independence whenever possible, even gradually. Rather than doing things for the patient, the caregiver adopts a supportive approach in which the patient is invited to participate as much as his or her abilities allow. For example, if a patient can only dress himself partially, the caregiver leaves it up to him to carry out the movements he can, intervening only where necessary. This method helps patients to regain control over their daily lives, which is essential for rebuilding their self-esteem.

In this approach, it is crucial to **value every effort** made by the patient, no matter how small. For a patient undergoing rehabilitation, accomplishing a task that used to be easy can now represent a real challenge. The caregiver must recognize the importance of any progress, no matter how small. For example, a patient who manages to stand up on his own after several weeks of immobility should be praised and encouraged. This appreciation of progress helps to boost the patient's self-confidence, showing him or her that he or she is capable of achieving goals and moving towards greater autonomy. This positive reinforcement is essential to motivate patients to continue their efforts and overcome their limitations, whether physical or psychological.

Another important aspect of rebuilding self-esteem is **the emotional** support the caregiver provides on a daily basis. Loss of autonomy can make some patients feel ashamed or guilty, especially those who were very independent before their hospitalization or accident. In these fragile moments, the caregiver must adopt a benevolent and reassuring attitude, reminding the patient that rehabilitation is a gradual process, and that each person progresses at his or her own pace. By listening empathetically and responding sympathetically to the patient's fears, the caregiver helps to relieve the emotional burden often associated with loss of autonomy.

Encouraging decision-making also plays a key role in rebuilding independence and self-esteem. One of the things that most affects self-esteem after a disabling event is the feeling of losing control over one's own life. By involving the patient in the decisions that concern him or her, even with regard to simple aspects of daily life, the caregiver enables the patient to regain a form of decision-making autonomy. For example, patients can choose the order of their day's activities, decide when they want to do their rehabilitation exercises, or opt for tasks they wish to carry out alone. These decisions, albeit minor, restore the patient's sense of control and boost their confidence in their own abilities.

The caregiver must also adapt care and assistance to the patient's **evolving abilities**. It is important to know how to gradually reduce the level of assistance as the patient regains strength and mobility. For example, a patient starting to walk with the aid of a walker may need constant support at first, but the caregiver must be prepared to lighten this assistance as the patient progresses. By encouraging this gradual autonomy, the caregiver enables the patient to see his or her own improvement and regain confidence in his or her physical abilities, while ensuring that safety is always guaranteed.

In addition, the caregiver can encourage the patient to **set personal goals** that are meaningful to him or her. These may be tasks they wish to accomplish themselves, such as preparing a meal, getting fully dressed, or even going out for a walk. By defining realistic, personalized goals with the patient, the caregiver helps him or her to look to the future and give meaning to daily efforts. Achieving these goals, however modest, helps to boost self-esteem, as patients regain a sense of control over important aspects of their lives.

The importance of self-esteem is not limited to the physical aspects of rehabilitation, but also affects psychological and social well-being. The caregiver can encourage the patient to maintain social ties, whether with family, friends or other rehab patients. Social interaction is a key element in rebuilding self-esteem, as it enables the patient to feel integrated, listened to and supported. By encouraging these exchanges, the caregiver helps the patient to regain an active place in his or her environment, helping to improve self-image and restore confidence.

Finally, the caregiver's **patience and perseverance** are indispensable in this reconstruction process. Each patient progresses at his or her own pace, and it is important to respect this timeframe, without rushing progress or imposing unrealistic expectations. By adapting to the patient's individual needs, the caregiver shows that he or she is there to support without judging, creating a framework conducive to the re-emergence of self-confidence and independence.

Chapter 5

Specific pathologies and their impact on rehabilitation

Stroke and neurological rehabilitation

- The caregiver's role in motor and cognitive recovery.

The role of the caregiver in the motor and cognitive recovery of patients is both fundamental and versatile. In a rehabilitation context, where patients are striving to regain physical and mental capacities that are sometimes severely impaired, the caregiver is at the heart of the recovery process. They work closely with other healthcare professionals, such as physiotherapists, occupational therapists and doctors, and play a key role in the day-to-day care of patients. Their work extends far beyond basic care: they are directly involved in encouraging and supporting patients in their efforts to regain their mobility, coordination and cognitive faculties, while fostering their motivation and self-confidence.

When it comes to **motor recovery**, the caregiver plays an essential supporting role. After an accident or surgery, or as a result of neurological or degenerative diseases, many patients find their ability to move limited. The caregiver's constant presence and daily interactions help patients with simple but crucial tasks. For example, they help them to get up, to walk with technical aids, or to carry out specific movements prescribed by physiotherapists. By helping patients perform these movements, the caregiver ensures that the exercises are carried out correctly, safely and, above all, without risking further injury.

This **assistance with mobilization** goes hand in hand with constant monitoring of the patient's progress. The caregiver observes changes in muscle strength, endurance and balance, while identifying any difficulties encountered by the patient. If signs of excessive fatigue, pain or exhaustion appear, he or she immediately adjusts the intensity of movements or informs the medical team of the need to reassess the rehabilitation program. This vigilance helps to ensure appropriate progress and prevent relapses or complications, while helping to adapt the rehabilitation program to the patient's current capabilities.

The caregiver's support is not limited to prescribed exercises: he or she is also involved in everyday activities. By helping the patient to **relearn the movements of everyday life**, such as standing up, bending over or even getting dressed, the caregiver integrates motor rehabilitation into daily care. This enables the patient to assimilate these movements more quickly into his or her routine, making progress more concrete and directly applicable to regaining autonomy.

The caregiver's role also extends to **cognitive recovery**, especially for patients with neurological disorders such as stroke, head injury or certain neurodegenerative diseases. In these cases, cognitive functions such as memory, concentration, language and organizational skills can be impaired. The caregiver assists patients with cognitive rehabilitation, facilitating their participation in mental stimulation exercises proposed by occupational therapists and neuropsychologists. For example, they can help patients to follow instructions, concentrate on specific tasks, or perform memory exercises. These activities, though sometimes simple, make a major contribution to rebuilding cognitive functions.

Day-to-day cognitive stimulation is also a fundamental aspect of the caregiver's role. By engaging patients in discussions, asking them questions to stimulate their memory, or inviting them to take part in playful or intellectual activities, the caregiver helps to maintain and improve the patient's cognitive abilities. This informal but regular approach is essential, as it enables the brain to be stimulated in a natural way, within the framework of normal social interactions, thus promoting progressive and less formal cognitive rehabilitation.

The caregiver also plays an important role in **adapting the environment** to the patient's motor and cognitive abilities. In collaboration with the rehabilitation team, he/she ensures that the patient's environment is safe and adapted to his/her specific needs. This may include installing grab bars, ergonomic cushions, or adapting the space to facilitate movement. The environment thus becomes an active rehabilitation tool, enabling patients to move around more easily and concentrate on recovering their functions without putting themselves at risk. By ensuring the patient's safety and comfort, the caregiver helps to create an environment conducive to rehabilitation, where every movement and every action reinforces progress.

Another important aspect of the caregiver's role in motor and cognitive recovery is **psychological encouragement**. Recovery, whether physical or cognitive, is often long and fraught with moments of frustration. Some patients may lose hope or become discouraged by slow progress. The caregiver, through his or her daily presence, plays an essential moral support role. They value small steps forward, even when they seem insignificant, and remind the patient that every step counts in the overall rehabilitation process. By offering regular encouragement and maintaining a positive attitude, the caregiver helps to keep the patient motivated, a key factor in successful recovery.

Finally, the caregiver works closely with the entire care team to adjust and refine recovery strategies. They communicate regularly with physiotherapists, occupational therapists and doctors, informing them of the patient's progress or difficulties. This fluid communication makes it possible to reassess rehabilitation objectives and ensure that the care plan remains adapted to the patient's evolving needs. The caregiver's observations and daily involvement provide invaluable information that helps to adjust care in real time.

- Challenges specific to patients suffering from aphasia or paralysis.

Patients suffering from aphasia or paralysis present specific challenges that require an adapted and caring approach on the part of the caregiver. Aphasia, which affects the ability to communicate verbally following a stroke or brain injury, and paralysis, which results in partial or total loss of mobility, disrupt patients' daily lives and have a major impact on their autonomy. Faced with these conditions, the caregiver plays a crucial role in supporting the patient, both in managing physical limitations and communication difficulties, and in the rehabilitation process, offering personalized, empathetic support.

The first challenge for patients suffering from **aphasia** is the difficulty in **expressing their needs** and understanding the information communicated to them. Aphasia can impair the ability to speak, understand, read or write, depending on the severity and type of aphasia. This creates a sense of frustration and isolation for patients, who are often aware of what they want to say, but are unable to formulate it correctly. As caregivers are in direct contact with patients on a daily basis, they need to adapt their way of communicating to make exchanges as simple and comprehensible as possible. This means using short, clear sentences and non-verbal language, reinforced by gestures, facial expressions and visual demonstrations. For example, pointing to an object or showing an action can facilitate comprehension when an aphasic patient is unable to grasp oral instructions.

To help aphasic patients **express themselves**, caregivers can also encourage the use of **alternative communication tools**, such as pictograms, communication tablets or simple word cards. These devices enable the patient to choose images or words to indicate needs or express emotions. The use of these tools helps to reduce the sense of frustration associated with the inability to express oneself verbally, while maintaining a certain level of independence in communication. The caregiver must be patient and encourage the patient to take his or her time in making himself or herself understood, while valuing every attempt at communication, however modest.

Emotional support is also crucial for aphasic patients, who may feel isolated, misunderstood, or lose confidence because of their communication difficulties. The caregiver must establish a climate of trust, showing empathy and taking the time to listen actively, even if the conversation is slow or difficult. It's essential that the patient feels that his or her efforts to communicate are valued and respected. This attention and caring helps to reduce the patient's anxiety and reinforce his or her motivation to participate actively in rehabilitation.

Patients suffering from **paralysis** face major physical challenges, particularly in terms of **mobility** and **independence in daily activities**. Paralysis may be partial or total, affecting one or more limbs, and severely limiting the patient's ability to move independently, dress, wash or eat. The caregiver must therefore be constantly attentive to the needs of these patients, providing them with appropriate physical support while seeking to preserve their autonomy as far as possible. For example, it may be necessary to help a patient make safe transfers from bed to wheelchair, or to accompany them in their movements using technical aids such as walkers or grab bars.

In this context, one of the challenges for the caregiver is to strike a balance between **providing assistance and encouraging autonomy**. It is crucial not to do everything for the patient that he or she could do alone, even partially, as this could slow down rehabilitation. For example, a patient paralyzed in one arm can still learn to use the other arm for certain tasks, such as eating or washing. The caregiver must encourage these autonomous gestures, providing support only when necessary, while ensuring that the patient is safe.

Another challenge for paralyzed patients is the **prevention of complications associated with immobility**, such as pressure sores and muscle contractures. Caregivers must be particularly vigilant to these risks, and regularly reposition the patient to prevent prolonged pressure points from causing skin lesions. Passive mobilization - the gentle movement of paralyzed limbs to keep joints supple - is also an essential task. This daily attention helps prevent complications, while maintaining a minimum of movement in the paralyzed limbs.

Paralyzed patients can also experience **psychological difficulties** linked to loss of mobility and dependence. Losing the ability to move freely and perform simple tasks can lead to feelings of frustration, worthlessness and sometimes depression. The caregiver must be aware of these psychological issues and provide constant emotional support. This means listening to the patient, acknowledging the small progress he or she has made, and creating a respectful, caring environment. It is essential to remind the patient that rehabilitation is a long process, but that each step, however small, is a step towards improvement.

Another important aspect is **adapting the environment** to make life easier for patients with aphasia or paralysis. The caregiver, in collaboration with the rehabilitation team, must ensure that the patient's living space is designed to maximize independence and reduce the risk of falls or injury. For example, in the case of paralyzed patients, this may include installing grab bars in the bathroom, using adapted shower chairs, or arranging the bed so that it's easier to get in and out of. For aphasic patients, the presence of visual aids or communication aids in their immediate environment can make daily life easier.

Post-operative rehabilitation: Orthopedic and cardio-respiratory surgery

- Supporting patients who have undergone prostheses, complex fractures or coronary bypass surgery.

Caring for patients who have undergone prostheses, complex fractures or coronary bypass surgery represents a major challenge for caregivers, as these procedures touch on profound physical and psychological aspects. Not only do these patients have to cope with post-operative pain and the demands of rehabilitation, but they are often also faced with fears and doubts about their ability to return to a normal life. The role of the caregiver in this context is essential, as he or she is on the front line in helping patients overcome the difficulties of recovery and guiding them step by step towards regained autonomy. The caregiver's role is to provide both physical and moral support, restoring the patient's confidence in his or her own body and offering constant support.

For patients who have had **prostheses** fitted, whether to the hip, knee or shoulder, rehabilitation is an unavoidable and often trying stage. The body has to adapt to the presence of this new element, and the patient has to relearn how to move, walk and perform everyday tasks. From the very first post-operative days, the caregiver helps with mobilization, scrupulously respecting medical recommendations, particularly in terms of movements to be avoided. For example, in the case of a hip prosthesis, certain movements, such as bending the hip excessively or crossing the legs, are prohibited to avoid the risk of dislocation. The caregiver helps the patient to stand up, walk with crutches or a walker, ensuring that these movements are made safely and in the correct posture.

One of the major challenges for these patients is **pain management**. After a prosthesis has been fitted, pain can be intense, discouraging the patient from undertaking the rehabilitation exercises necessary for recovery. The caregiver, through his or her daily support, plays a key role in encouraging the patient to pursue rehabilitation despite the pain. They also ensure that the pace of exercise is adapted to the patient's condition, while alerting the nursing team to any unusual intensification of pain. The aim is to strike a balance between relieving pain and maintaining progressive mobilization to avoid joint stiffness or post-operative complications.

Valuing progress is also essential for these patients. Every stage of rehabilitation, no matter how small, must be acknowledged and encouraged. For example, if a patient manages to walk a few extra metres every day with a hip or knee prosthesis, the caregiver should congratulate the patient on his or her efforts, thereby boosting confidence and encouraging perseverance. Moral support is just as important as physical support, because the rehabilitation process can be long and fraught with moments of discouragement.

For patients with **complex fractures**, rehabilitation is often more difficult and time-consuming, especially if the fracture necessitated surgery involving the installation of hardware (plates, screws, nails). These fractures can affect highly stressed areas of the body, such as the arms or legs, and the patient must learn to mobilize the injured areas while respecting precautionary instructions. The caregiver must be vigilant about how the patient performs the first movements, to avoid excessive stress on the healing fracture. He or she helps the patient to gently mobilize the affected area, performing progressive muscle-strengthening exercises, while ensuring that the patient does not exceed his or her physical limits.

Psychological support is just as important here. Patients who have suffered complex fractures can sometimes be severely limited in their autonomy for several weeks or months, which can be a source of frustration and discouragement. The caregiver needs to listen to these emotions and offer constant moral support, reminding the patient that recovery is a gradual process. By rewarding every small improvement, such as increased mobility or reduced pain, the caregiver helps to reinforce the patient's motivation.

For patients who have undergone **coronary bypass** surgery, the stakes are both physical and psychological. This operation, often performed as an emergency or after serious episodes such as heart attacks, plunges the patient into a situation where he or she has to relearn how to manage his or her body, physical exertion and stress. Convalescence after bypass surgery requires special attention, as the patient must gradually resume physical activities while avoiding excessive strain on the heart. The caregiver plays a key role in monitoring the patient's general condition, checking vital constants (blood pressure, heart rate) and ensuring that the first movements, such as standing up or walking, are carried out safely.

One of the greatest challenges for these patients is to regain **confidence in their physical abilities** after cardiac surgery. Many of them are afraid to use their heart or exert themselves, for fear of provoking another attack. The caregiver, in collaboration with the medical team, must encourage the patient to gradually resume appropriate physical activity, while reassuring them that such efforts are not only safe, but necessary to strengthen the heart. For example, walking short distances or doing breathing exercises to improve lung capacity are important steps towards regaining physical fitness. The caregiver ensures that these activities are carried out gradually and in a safe environment.

Cardiac rehabilitation, often prescribed after bypass surgery, is a process that involves both physical exercise and education in stress and lifestyle management. The caregiver can help the patient to adopt healthy habits on a daily basis, whether by monitoring his or her diet, encouraging him or her to respect rest and exercise guidelines, or helping him or her to manage anxiety linked to the condition. This comprehensive approach, which combines physical and psychological aspects, enables patients to regain a balance between activity and rest, while learning to take better care of their heart.

- Specific monitoring and management of post-operative complications.

Specific monitoring and management of post-operative complications are essential aspects of the nursing auxiliary's work, particularly in rehabilitation and intensive care units. After surgery, the patient's body is in a recovery and healing phase, but it is also vulnerable to a number of potential complications, both immediate and delayed. The caregiver, through his or her daily presence and careful observation, plays a key role in the early detection of these complications and their rapid management, in collaboration with the nursing team. This vigilance ensures that the healing process proceeds in the best possible conditions, and that the patient's state of health does not worsen.

The first step in **postoperative monitoring** is regular monitoring of the patient's **vital signs**, such as body temperature, blood pressure, pulse and respiratory rate. Any abnormal variation in these parameters may indicate a complication. For example, a high fever may indicate a postoperative infection, while a drop in blood pressure or a rapid pulse may signal internal bleeding. By carefully monitoring and recording these vitals, the caregiver helps to detect early warning signs that require immediate medical intervention. In the event of any abnormality, the caregiver quickly alerts the medical team, enabling action to be taken before the situation worsens.

Surgical wound monitoring is also an essential component of postoperative care. Wounds, whether closed with sutures or staples, or left open to heal, must be monitored regularly for signs of infection, inflammation or bleeding. The caregiver checks the appearance of the wound, the cleanliness of the dressing, and the presence of any redness, warmth, purulent discharge or unusual odor. If there is any suspicion of infection or complication, such as dehiscence (spontaneous opening of the wound), the caregiver immediately alerts the nurse or doctor for further assessment and appropriate treatment.

Postoperative **respiratory** complications, such as atelectasis or pneumonia, are common, particularly in bedridden patients or those who have undergone major surgery. Caregivers must be alert to these risks and encourage patients to perform breathing exercises, such as deep breathing or the use of an incentive spirometer, to maintain good lung ventilation and prevent secretion build-up. By monitoring the patient's breathing, the caregiver can identify signs of shortness of breath, shallow breathing or chest pain, which require prompt attention to prevent a deterioration in respiratory status.

Another common complication is **deep vein thrombosis (DVT)**, which can occur in bedridden patients or those with reduced mobility. DVT involves the formation of blood clots, usually in the legs, and can progress to pulmonary embolism, which is potentially fatal. The caregiver must be alert to signs of thrombosis, such as swelling of the lower limbs, redness or localized pain. He or she may also encourage the patient to perform leg mobilization exercises to stimulate blood circulation, or ensure that devices such as compression stockings or intermittent compression systems are used correctly. In addition to visual monitoring, the caregiver's role is to remind the patient of the importance of early mobilization, even passive mobilization, to reduce the risk of clot formation.

Post-operative **digestive complications**, such as constipation, nausea or vomiting, are also common concerns. They can result from the side effects of drugs (especially opioids), anesthesia or immobility. The caregiver must monitor the patient's bowel habits and report any signs of bowel obstruction, such as a prolonged absence of bowel movements or severe abdominal pain. In collaboration with the medical team, they can suggest measures to prevent these complications, such as administering mild laxatives, promoting hydration, or encouraging mobilization to promote intestinal transit.

Urinary complications, such as urine retention or urinary tract infection, are also to be monitored, especially in patients who have been catheterized during the procedure or immediately afterwards. The caregiver must ensure that the patient urinates regularly and painlessly, and observe any signs of infection, such as pain on urination, abnormal urine color or the presence of blood. In the case of a urinary catheter, he or she must also check that the catheter is functioning correctly, without obstruction, and that hygiene measures are scrupulously observed to minimize the risk of infection.

Psychological support is another important aspect of post-operative monitoring. After surgery, some patients may experience anxiety, depression or confusion, particularly after general anaesthesia or in the elderly. The caregiver's proximity and attentiveness can detect signs of emotional distress or disorientation and act accordingly. By offering an attentive ear, gently explaining care and reassuring the patient about the healing process, the caregiver helps to allay fears and support the patient's emotional state, thus promoting better recovery.

In addition, the caregiver must be attentive to **postoperative pain management**. Poorly managed pain can slow recovery, disrupt sleep, and make the patient reluctant to move, increasing the risk of complications such as pressure sores or DVT. By monitoring pain intensity using appropriate scales, and ensuring that analgesic treatments are administered appropriately, the caregiver plays a key role in patient comfort. If pain persists or becomes unbearable despite treatment, it is essential to inform the medical team promptly so that doses can be adjusted or other methods of relief suggested, such as physiotherapy or relaxation techniques.

Finally, **early mobilization** of the patient, when authorized by the medical team, is a key element in postoperative recovery. The caregiver helps the patient to get up gradually, to walk and to change position, while ensuring that these movements are carried out in complete safety. Mobilization helps to improve blood circulation, reduce the risk of respiratory and digestive complications, and promote faster recovery. The caregiver must encourage this regular activity, adapted to the patient's abilities, and offer constant support to avoid falls or sudden movements that could aggravate pain or cause injury.

Patients suffering from chronic illnesses: diabetes, kidney failure, etc.
- How to adapt care and exercise to chronic pathologies.

Adapting care and exercise to patients with chronic pathologies is a complex challenge that requires an individualized and nuanced approach. Chronic diseases such as diabetes, cardiovascular disease, respiratory conditions such as COPD, or degenerative diseases such as multiple sclerosis or osteoarthritis, directly influence patients' ability to participate in care and rehabilitation. For each patient, the chronicity of their pathology requires constant adjustment of care, to respect their physical limits and prevent symptoms from worsening, while seeking to maintain or improve their quality of life.

The first step in adapting care is a **thorough understanding of the** patient's **pathology** and its specific manifestations. Each chronic disease presents a different clinical picture, and each patient reacts uniquely to his or her condition. It is therefore essential for the caregiver, in collaboration with the medical team, to take into account the physical limitations and pain associated with the pathology. For example, a patient suffering from osteoarthritis will have joint pain that limits mobility, while a patient with a chronic respiratory disease such as COPD will quickly become short of breath on exertion. Adapting care to these realities means listening to the patient, respecting his or her current capabilities, and not forcing movements or exercises that could aggravate symptoms.

In the case of patients suffering from **chronic pain**, such as osteoarthritis or musculoskeletal pathologies, care and exercise must be adapted to the patient's pain threshold. Rehabilitation exercises should aim **to maintain joint mobility and strengthen muscles** without exacerbating pain. The caregiver can encourage gentle, progressive movements, such as low-impact range-of-motion exercises or light stretching. For example, for a patient suffering from osteoarthritis of the knee, passive mobilization of the joint or exercises in a seated or lying position may be more appropriate than an activity that places heavy demands on weight-bearing joints, such as walking. The aim is to avoid complete inactivity, which can aggravate stiffness and pain, while respecting the limits imposed by pain.

Patients suffering from **chronic respiratory illnesses**, such as COPD or severe asthma, require special attention in managing their breathlessness and respiratory capacity. The caregiver must ensure that physical exercises are adapted to the patient's effort tolerance, taking care not to provoke attacks of dyspnea. Breathing exercises, such as abdominal breathing or the use of an incentive spirometer, can be incorporated into the daily routine to strengthen lung capacity and improve ventilation. These exercises help reduce the sensation of breathlessness and prevent respiratory infections by promoting the evacuation of secretions. It is essential for the caregiver to remain vigilant to the patient's respiratory status during exercise, watching for signs such as excessive breathlessness, cyanosis or rapid, shallow breathing, and adjusting exercises accordingly.

For patients with **chronic cardiovascular disease**, such as heart failure or post-myocardial infarction, care and exercise must be carefully balanced. The aim is to gradually improve the patient's physical capacity without overloading the heart. The caregiver, in liaison with the rehabilitation team, helps to set up light exercises, such as slow walking or low-intensity muscle-strengthening activities. These exercises aim to improve endurance without causing cardiac stress. It's crucial to watch for signs of excessive fatigue, such as shortness of breath, chest pain or unusual sweating. If in doubt, the caregiver should stop the exercise and consult the medical team. Cardiac rehabilitation also involves educating patients on how to manage their daily effort, and the caregiver plays a key role in providing practical advice on stress management, healthy living and eating habits.

Diabetic patients, especially those with type 2 diabetes, require special management of blood sugar levels during care and exercise. The caregiver must ensure that exercise is appropriate and does not cause sudden variations in blood glucose levels, either hypoglycemia or hyperglycemia. Before starting any physical activity, it is essential to measure the patient's blood sugar level and ensure that it is within a safe range. During exercise, the caregiver watches for signs of hypoglycemia, such as tremors, sudden fatigue, confusion or cold sweats. It is also important to advise the patient on the importance of maintaining a balanced diet before and after exercise, to avoid excessive glycemic variations. Exercise for diabetic patients should be moderate, such as walking, stretching or water exercises, to help regulate blood sugar levels without causing undue stress on the body.

For patients suffering from **neurodegenerative pathologies** such as multiple sclerosis or Parkinson's disease, adapting care and exercises is essential to preserve mobility while taking account of fluctuating symptoms. These diseases are often characterized by periods of remission and relapses, and the caregiver must adapt care to the patient's condition at each stage. In relapse phases, when symptoms are more severe (e.g. tremors, muscle spasms, severe fatigue), care must be aimed at maintaining comfort and preventing complications associated with immobility, such as bedsores or urinary tract infections. Exercise during these periods should be limited to gentle mobilization and prevention of joint stiffness. In phases of remission, the caregiver can encourage more active activities, always adapted to the patient's abilities, to maintain muscle strength, coordination and balance.

Adapting care not only concerns physical rehabilitation, but also the **management of other aspects of daily life**. For a patient suffering from a chronic illness, even simple gestures can become difficult. The caregiver must ensure that these gestures are carried out in the best possible conditions, using technical aids if necessary. For example, a patient suffering from rheumatoid arthritis may find it difficult to feed or dress himself, due to stiffness and joint pain. In this case, the caregiver can suggest adapted utensils, such as ergonomic cutlery or easy-to-slip-on clothing, to maintain a degree of independence despite the disease.

- The link between rehabilitation and the prevention of chronic disease complications.

The link between rehabilitation and the prevention of complications associated with chronic diseases is essential to improve patients' quality of life and prevent their health from worsening. Chronic illnesses such as diabetes, heart failure, respiratory diseases such as COPD, and osteoarthritis require long-term management, not only to treat symptoms, but also to prevent potential complications that can seriously impact a patient's autonomy and overall health. Rehabilitation plays a central role here, helping to maintain and even improve physical and functional capacities, while reducing the risks associated with these pathologies.

One of the fundamental links between rehabilitation and the prevention of complications is that rehabilitation helps **maintain mobility and muscle strength**, which is essential for preventing complications associated with immobility. In patients suffering from chronic diseases, prolonged inactivity, often caused by pain or fatigue, can lead to loss of muscle mass, reduced joint flexibility and, ultimately, loss of autonomy. This can lead to a vicious circle in which reduced mobility worsens the patient's condition and increases the risk of falls, fractures and respiratory complications. By incorporating regular exercise tailored to each patient's abilities, rehabilitation helps maintain physical activity, prevent joint stiffness and strengthen muscles. For example, for a patient suffering from osteoarthritis, low-impact exercises such as walking or swimming help to keep joints supple, while reducing pain and maintaining muscle strength.

Similarly, in chronic diseases such as **COPD or severe asthma**, respiratory rehabilitation is crucial to prevent serious respiratory complications. Patients with chronic respiratory diseases are at risk of developing lung infections, such as pneumonia, due to the accumulation of secretions and weakness of respiratory muscles. Breathing exercises, such as diaphragmatic breathing or the use of pulmonary expansion devices, promote better lung ventilation, prevent bronchial congestion and reduce the frequency of disease exacerbations. In addition, rehabilitation helps improve exercise capacity, reducing breathlessness and enabling patients to remain active for longer without excessive respiratory discomfort.

In the case **of cardiovascular diseases**, such as heart failure or post-myocardial infarction, cardiac rehabilitation plays a fundamental role in preventing complications. A sedentary lifestyle in these patients increases the risk of recurrence of serious cardiac events, such as heart attacks or strokes. Rehabilitation exercises, carried out under medical supervision, aim to strengthen cardiac capacity and improve endurance. By following a progressive, moderate exercise program, such as walking or gentle muscle-strengthening exercises, patients can reduce their blood pressure, improve circulation and strengthen their heart, while reducing the risk of complications. What's more, rehabilitation also offers an opportunity for education in stress management, anxiety and the adoption of healthy lifestyles, which are key elements in the prevention of cardiovascular disease.

The link between rehabilitation and the prevention of complications is also strong in **diabetes management**. In diabetic patients, particularly those with type 2 diabetes, physical rehabilitation is an indispensable tool for improving insulin sensitivity and promoting better glycemic control. By stimulating the muscles, physical activity helps the body to use glucose more efficiently, thereby regulating blood sugar levels. What's more, rehabilitation helps prevent the frequent complications of diabetes, such as peripheral neuropathy, infections and circulatory problems. By maintaining regular physical activity, diabetic patients reduce the risk of developing foot ulcers and other complications linked to poor circulation. In addition, physical exercise also promotes weight management, a crucial factor in controlling diabetes and preventing the complications associated with obesity.

Preventing psychological complications is another central aspect of rehabilitating patients suffering from chronic illnesses. These long-term conditions, particularly when they impair autonomy, can lead to disorders such as depression, anxiety and feelings of hopelessness. By integrating both physical and psychological aspects, rehabilitation helps to combat social isolation and strengthen patients' mental well-being. By actively participating in rehabilitation programs, patients can regain a sense of control over their body and condition, which is crucial to maintaining good mental health. The caregiver, by providing guidance and moral support, also plays a key role in preventing these complications, by valuing progress and creating an environment conducive to the patient's psychological development.

Last but not least, rehabilitation offers a **comprehensive, educational approach** that helps prevent the complications of chronic illnesses in the long term. Rehabilitation programs are not limited to physical exercise: they also include therapeutic education aimed at teaching patients how to manage their disease on a daily basis. Whether it's a heart patient learning to recognize the warning signs of an attack, a diabetic learning to manage his or her blood sugar levels according to diet and physical activity, or an asthma patient receiving advice on how to manage attacks, this education is an essential pillar in the prevention of complications. The caregiver, in collaboration with the medical team, reinforces this educational dimension with daily reminders of the importance of respecting care, monitoring and lifestyle instructions.

Chapter 6

Managing young and pediatric rehabilitation patients

Special care for children
- Adapting care and communication to the needs of children in rehabilitation.

Adapting care and communication to the needs of children undergoing rehabilitation is both a technical and emotional challenge, because caring for these young patients requires a specific approach, adapted to their age, level of development and physical and psychological state. Children undergoing rehabilitation, whether they have undergone surgery, suffered a trauma or have a chronic pathology, have a very different experience from adults. They may experience fears, misunderstandings and a sense of loss of control, making emotional support as important as physical care. The caregiver plays a central role in adapting care and communicating with these young patients, in order to reassure them, motivate them and help them regain their physical abilities and self-confidence.

One of the first adaptations needed is to **personalize care** according to the child's age and level of development. A young child does not have the same understanding of illness, the body or pain as an adolescent. The caregiver must therefore adjust his or her approach according to the child's cognitive abilities. For example, with a young child, care must be presented in a simple, reassuring way, using explanations adapted to the child's vocabulary and comprehension. It's also important to use gentle gestures, to warn the child before any medical procedure, and to incorporate playful elements to make the experience less intimidating. For a teenager, communication can be more direct, taking care to involve the child in decisions that concern him or her, and respecting his or her need for autonomy.

Another fundamental aspect of adapting care is **pain management**. Children, especially the youngest, may find it difficult to express precisely what they are feeling, and pain assessment can be difficult. The caregiver needs to be alert to non-verbal signs, such as crying, grimacing, agitation or isolation, which may indicate pain or discomfort. The use of adapted assessment tools, such as face scales for younger children, helps to better understand the intensity of pain and to adjust care accordingly. The caregiver must also explain to the child, in a simple and reassuring way, the measures put in place to relieve pain, whether these involve medication or relaxation techniques. This helps reduce pain-related anxiety and helps the child tolerate pain better.

Communication with children in rehabilitation needs to be clear, reassuring and adapted to their level of understanding. Children often need to know what's going to happen to them to feel safe, but it's crucial to use language that isn't frightening. For example, rather than talking about an "injection" or "drip", terms like "a little medicine in your arm" or "a little shot that will help you feel better" may be more appropriate. The caregiver must always ensure that the child understands what is going to happen, while avoiding overloading him/her with information that could generate fear. The use of metaphors or role-playing can also be useful in explaining certain care procedures in a more playful, less anxiety-provoking way.

To help children feel involved in their own rehabilitation, it's important to give them **an active role** in their care. Even if the child is young, the caregiver can encourage him to participate as much as possible in his rehabilitation, by giving him simple choices, such as deciding on the order of exercises or choosing an exercise he prefers. This approach reinforces the child's sense of autonomy and control, both of which are crucial to improving adherence to the rehabilitation process. By involving the child, the caregiver shows him that his efforts are valued and that he has a key role to play in his own recovery.

Play and creativity are also powerful tools to help children **accept and participate in care**. Games, stories and distractions can divert the child's attention from difficult or painful moments and make the experience more enjoyable. For example, during a physical rehabilitation session, the caregiver can turn an exercise into a game, by challenging the child to walk to a specific point or by suggesting that he or she pretend to fly like a superhero during a stretching movement. This kind of playful approach helps keep the child engaged and motivated, while making care less stressful.

Emotional support is just as important. Children, especially the very young, may feel fear, frustration or sadness at their illness or temporary incapacity. The caregiver must show empathy, listening to the child's fears and reassuring him or her with simple, kind words. It's essential to acknowledge the child's emotions, telling him that it's normal to be scared or sad, while encouraging him to express his feelings. This emotional support is crucial in calming the child's anxiety and giving him the strength to overcome the obstacles of rehabilitation.

The **relationship with parents** is another fundamental aspect of supporting children in rehabilitation. Parents, too, are in a difficult situation and may be worried about their child, sometimes feeling powerless in the face of their child's suffering or limitations. The caregiver must include parents in the care process, explaining what is happening, answering their questions and reassuring them about their child's progress. It's important to establish a bond of trust with parents, as their support and involvement in rehabilitation are essential to the success of the process. By involving them, the caregiver helps to strengthen the bond between child and family, creating a coherent, caring environment.

Lastly, the caregiver must take care to **adapt physical care** to the specific needs of children, taking into account their size, strength and stamina. Rehabilitation exercises, whether aimed at improving mobility, muscular strength or coordination, must be adapted to the child's age and physical capabilities. For example, a child who has suffered a fracture or undergone surgery will require progressive, light exercises at first, before gradually increasing the intensity as the child progresses. It's essential to respect the child's rhythm, without pushing him beyond his limits, while encouraging him to continue his efforts with gentleness and patience.

- The role of the caregiver in supporting psychomotor development.

The role of the caregiver in supporting the psychomotor development of patients, particularly children and the elderly, is essential in promoting the harmonious evolution of physical and mental capacities. Psychomotor development concerns the interaction between motor functions (such as movement coordination, balance and posture) and psychological functions (such as perception, attention, memory and emotional management). In children, appropriate support promotes the healthy growth of these crucial skills, while in the elderly or in rehabilitation patients, this support helps to maintain or regain these abilities after an accident or illness.

One of the caregiver's first tasks in this context is to **stimulate motor skills**, while taking into account each patient's individual abilities. In children, the development of fine and gross motor skills is a natural process, but it can be slowed or compromised by developmental delays, illness or accidents. The caregiver supports the child by proposing age-appropriate activities that encourage coordination and gesture control. For example, simple exercises such as catching a ball, balancing on a line, or handling small objects, help develop both coordination and dexterity. These activities should never be imposed, but encouraged in a playful way, so that children enjoy moving around and exploring their environment.

More generally, the caregiver plays a key role in **creating a stimulating and secure environment** in which the child or patient can develop both physically and psychologically. This means providing a setting where movement is encouraged, but also where the patient feels confident to take motor initiatives without fear of injury or failure. For children, this environment can include games that challenge both body and mind, such as puzzles or motor courses, which require the child to plan his or her movements and use concentration. For the elderly or those undergoing rehabilitation, this care environment must be safe to prevent falls, while remaining conducive to motor and cognitive stimulation, for example by creating spaces that encourage walking, stretching or the manipulation of simple objects.

Cognitive stimulation, which goes hand in hand with motor activities, is another major component of psychomotor support. Psychomotor development is based on the ability to coordinate actions with conscious thought. In the case of children, this can take the form of educational games where they have to manipulate objects while thinking, for example by stacking blocks according to a certain size or color logic. The caregiver can encourage these activities, which not only strengthen motor skills, but also stimulate cognitive functions such as memory and concentration. For adults in rehabilitation or the elderly, cognitive exercises can include simple but engaging tasks, such as memory games, object recognition exercises, or even everyday tasks that require coordinating gestures with thought, such as cooking or tidying up.

In managing psychomotor development, **observation is** an essential skill for the caregiver. By closely monitoring each patient's progress and difficulties, the caregiver can adjust care and activities to better meet individual needs. In a child, for example, delays in fine motor skills (such as difficulty holding a pencil or tying shoes) may require specific activities to strengthen hand-eye coordination. Similarly, in an elderly person or one undergoing rehabilitation, signs of muscular weakness or balance problems need to be taken into account, so that exercises can be adapted to strengthen these abilities without overtaxing them.

Motivation is another fundamental aspect of the caregiver's role in supporting psychomotor development. Whether in children or adults, motor and cognitive learning can be long and fraught with frustration. The caregiver plays a crucial role in encouraging patients to persevere, valuing each small step forward, and creating an atmosphere of support and encouragement. In children, this motivation can be achieved through playful approaches, such as turning an exercise into a game or proposing age-appropriate challenges, while taking care not to apply excessive pressure that could discourage them. For adults, especially those undergoing rehabilitation after an accident or operation, the caregiver must regularly remind them of the importance of these exercises in regaining their autonomy, while respecting each individual's own rhythm.

The caregiver must also take into account the **emotional aspect of** psychomotor development. In children in particular, the development of motor and cognitive skills is closely linked to the management of emotions. An anxious or stressed child will find it harder to concentrate or perform precise gestures. The caregiver must therefore offer emotional support, establishing a climate of trust in which the child feels listened to and understood. For adults undergoing rehabilitation, serious injuries or pathologies can provoke feelings of frustration or devaluation. In such cases, the caregiver must be attentive to these emotions and offer psychological support, valuing the patient's efforts and encouraging him or her to remain committed to the rehabilitation process.

Finally, the caregiver's role in supporting psychomotor development also includes **collaboration with other professionals**, such as physiotherapists, occupational therapists and psychomotor therapists. The caregiver ensures daily monitoring of the exercises prescribed by these specialists, while providing regular feedback on the patient's progress. This collaboration makes it possible to adjust the rehabilitation program and ensure that the objectives set are achieved progressively, while respecting the patient's abilities.

Supporting young adults and teenagers
- Take into account the identity and emotional issues of young patients.

Taking into account the identity and emotional issues of young patients is a crucial component of their care, particularly when they are going through periods of rehabilitation or prolonged treatment. In children and teenagers, illness or disability often occurs at a time when personal identity is in full construction. This is a period marked by the search for self, the development of social relationships, and a quest for autonomy and recognition. In this context, the onset of a health problem or the need for rehabilitation can upset these dynamics, generating profound emotional challenges. The caregiver, through his or her daily accompaniment, plays an essential role in helping young people through this ordeal, while supporting their personal and emotional development.

One of the first aspects to take into account is young people's **perception of** their own **identity**, particularly when faced with illness or loss of autonomy. A child or teenager undergoing rehabilitation may feel different from others, which can affect his or her self-esteem. Physical transformations or functional limitations due to pathology can lead young people to perceive their body as an obstacle, to feel vulnerable, or to fear being judged by their peers. By listening to these concerns, the caregiver must show great empathy and find the words to reassure the young patient of his or her value, beyond their physical condition. It is essential to encourage a positive view of oneself, emphasizing preserved abilities or progress made, and helping the child to focus on what he can achieve, rather than on his limitations.

Emotional support is particularly important at this stage, as young patients can be overwhelmed by conflicting emotions: fear of the future, frustration at the slow pace of recovery, or anger at not being able to lead a "normal" life like their peers. These emotions must be welcomed by the caregiver, who must create a climate of trust in which the child or adolescent feels free to express them without fear of being judged. Rather than minimizing the young patient's emotions, it is crucial to recognize their legitimacy, while proposing solutions to overcome them. For example, encouraging relaxation methods, playful activities or open discussion can help channel stress and alleviate anxiety.

Social relationships are another major identity issue for young patients. In adolescence in particular, interactions with peers play a central role in the construction of identity. Prolonged hospitalization, repeated re-education sessions or the management of a chronic illness can isolate the adolescent from his or her social group, accentuating a feeling of marginalization. The caregiver must be attentive to this risk of isolation and encourage, as far as possible, the continuity of social relationships. This can take the form of exchanges with family and friends, visits from relatives, or the use of technology to keep in touch with friends. Maintaining these social ties is essential to prevent young people from closing in on themselves, and to preserve their sense of belonging, which is a pillar of self-esteem.

Autonomy is another key issue for young people undergoing rehabilitation or treatment. Childhood and especially adolescence are periods when independence gradually becomes a priority. Illness or rehabilitation, by forcing the child or adolescent to depend on others for acts of daily living, can engender a feeling of loss of control and regression. As far as possible, the caregiver should encourage the young patient's autonomy, even in small everyday tasks. The aim is to enable the child or adolescent to take part in his or her care, to make choices about treatment or activities, and to actively involve him or her in the recovery process. This participatory approach helps to restore a sense of mastery and reinforces self-esteem, while preparing the young patient to resume a more autonomous life after convalescence.

Another essential aspect is adapting **communication**. Young patients, especially teenagers, can sometimes find it difficult to express their feelings or understand the extent of their medical situation. The caregiver needs to adopt clear, age-appropriate communication, while respecting the patient's need to understand what's happening without being overwhelmed with information. With younger patients, this may involve explaining care in a visual or playful way, while with teenagers, it's about treating them as active partners in their treatment, explaining frankly and respectfully what's at stake, while answering their questions.

Last but not least, it's crucial to **reward** even the smallest **advances.** Young patients, faced with physical and emotional challenges, need regular positive feedback to stay motivated. The caregiver must be attentive to the slightest improvement, whether it's progress in a rehabilitation exercise, calmer pain management or a simple gesture performed independently. By highlighting these successes, the caregiver helps the young person maintain a positive outlook on his or her rehabilitation journey, while boosting confidence in his or her ability to overcome difficulties.

- Helping young people recovering from illness to return to school or work.

Helping convalescing young people return to school or work is a crucial step in their recovery process. After a period of hospitalization or rehabilitation, whether following illness, accident or surgery, young patients are often faced with major challenges in re-establishing their place in society, and particularly in school or the workplace. This transition can be a source of anxiety, both for the young people themselves and for their families, and requires appropriate support to ensure that reintegration takes place under the best possible conditions. By providing both physical and emotional support, the caregiver plays an essential role in this delicate phase, in collaboration with the medical team, teachers and, if necessary, employers.

The first step in facilitating this reintegration is to **prepare the young person to resume a rhythm of life compatible with his or her school or professional commitments**. During convalescence, the young patient has often lost certain habits linked to his or her daily activities, such as getting up at a fixed time, managing a timetable or carrying out tasks independently. The caregiver, in collaboration with the family and the care team, must gradually encourage the young patient to return to a certain routine. This can start with small tasks, such as keeping to a regular meal schedule, organizing the day around simple activities, or resuming rehabilitation exercises at set times. This gradual reintroduction of a time frame helps to bridge the gap between the period of convalescence and the return to school or working life, while giving the young person back a sense of control over his or her day.

Secondly, the caregiver must **ensure that the young person's physical and cognitive capacities** are **sufficiently strengthened** to enable him or her to adapt to the demands of reintegration. For example, a young person who has suffered a fracture or undergone surgery needs to be helped to regain his or her mobility, so that he or she can resume activities such as moving around independently in the school or workplace, or carrying a schoolbag or work tools. For young people who have experienced cognitive complications, such as after a head injury, it is crucial to work on concentration, memory and the ability to process information. The caregiver can encourage exercises tailored to these needs, in collaboration with professionals such as occupational therapists or neuropsychologists, so that the young person regains the confidence needed to invest in his or her studies or work again.

A key aspect of reintegration is also the **management of any lingering physical or medical limitations**. Some young people recovering from injury may still have after-effects, or have specific needs, such as adjustments to their schedule or environment. The caregiver, in liaison with the medical team and the educators or employers, must ensure that these adaptations are put in place. For example, a student with mobility problems may need help getting around the school, extra breaks, or a modified workstation. Similarly, a young person needing regular care, such as insulin injections for diabetes or medication, must be able to receive it without disrupting his or her schedule. The caregiver helps to organize these arrangements, ensuring that the young person can evolve in an inclusive and secure environment, without feeling stigmatized by his or her condition.

Communication between the care team, teachers or employers, and the family is also essential to ensure a smooth transition. The caregiver often plays a mediating role in this process, passing on to teachers or professional supervisors the necessary information about the young person's state of health and any specific accommodations he or she may need. This helps avoid misunderstandings and ensures that reintegration takes place under optimum conditions. For example, in a school context, teachers need to be informed of the young person's possible limitations in terms of physical or cognitive effort, so that they can adapt expectations and assessments accordingly. Similarly, an employer needs to be aware of the specific needs of a recovering employee to ensure a gradual return to work.

Another fundamental aspect of support is **emotional support**. Resuming school or professional life after a long period of convalescence can generate a great deal of anxiety in young people. They may fear that they won't be able to keep up, that they won't live up to expectations, or that their peers or colleagues will perceive them differently because of their illness. The caregiver needs to listen to these fears and offer reassuring support, valuing the efforts already made and emphasizing the young person's ability to overcome challenges. It's also important to encourage strategies for managing stress, such as breathing techniques, regular breaks or moments of relaxation. The return to normal can be gradual, and it's crucial that the young person doesn't feel rushed or overwhelmed by overly high expectations.

Finally, the caregiver can encourage the young person to **strengthen his or her social ties**, which play a key role in successful reintegration. During the period of convalescence, the young person may have been isolated from friends or colleagues, which can increase the feeling of loneliness or marginalization on his or her return. The caregiver must help to re-establish these relationships, by facilitating contact with peers, encouraging participation in social or group activities, and helping to overcome the fear of others' gaze. It is important to remind the young person that, although his illness or convalescence may have created a parenthesis, he can resume his place in the group, and that his reintegration is a sign of strength and courage.

Support for parents and relatives of paediatric patients
- Manage parents' anxiety and involve them in care without overburdening them.

Managing parents' anxiety and involving them in their child's care, while avoiding overburdening them, is a delicate but essential balance in the care of young patients. When a child or teenager goes through a period of illness, convalescence or rehabilitation, parents are often overwhelmed by conflicting emotions: fear, helplessness, concern for their child's future, but also a strong desire to be involved in every aspect of care. Their involvement is important, as they play a crucial role in their child's emotional and psychological support, but it is equally important to protect them from emotional or physical exhaustion.

One of the first steps in managing parents' anxiety is to **provide them with clear, detailed information tailored to their needs**. Uncertainty is often the main source of anxiety. When parents don't fully understand their child's situation or upcoming procedures, their fear increases. The caregiver must therefore take the time to explain, in an accessible and empathetic way, the child's state of health, the stages of treatment or rehabilitation, and the long-term objectives. This explanation should be reassuring but honest, avoiding downplaying the challenges ahead, while emphasizing the resources and progress possible. It is also important to give parents the opportunity to ask questions and express their concerns, so as to include them fully in the care dynamic, while meeting their emotional needs.

Establishing a climate of trust between parents and the healthcare team is essential, as it goes a long way towards easing anxiety. When parents feel confident, they are more inclined to delegate part of the care to the medical team, which relieves them of some of the pressure. The caregiver, through his or her daily presence and role as mediator, must be a point of reference for parents. By creating a relationship based on transparency and empathy, he or she helps parents understand that their child is in good hands, reducing their sense of helplessness. For example, by regularly checking in with parents, informing them of any progress made, however small, or explaining the care their child is receiving, the caregiver reassures them while enabling them to stay connected to the situation without becoming overwhelmed.

Another key aspect is **defining their role in care**. It's natural for parents to want to be as involved as possible in their child's care, but this involvement needs to be supervised to prevent them from feeling overwhelmed. The caregiver should encourage parents to take part in activities that strengthen the bond with their child, such as accompanying them in certain simple exercises or participating in moments of relaxation and emotional support, while sparing them from more technical or medical tasks, which are the responsibility of the care team. For example, a parent may be invited to help their child with play or educational activities adapted to their condition, or to support them during moments of gentle exercise, but more complex care (such as dressings or monitoring vitals) must be handled by professionals. This allows parents to be present in a positive way, without having to bear the full burden of medical care.

At the same time, it is essential to **recognize and value their role** in the emotional and psychological care of their child. Parents are often the best emotional support for their children. They can play a vital role in providing reassurance, encouragement and emotional support on a daily basis. The caregiver should remind them that, even if they are not directly involved in all medical care, their simple presence, love and emotional support are essential to their child's morale and recovery. For example, moments of complicity, soothing discussions, gestures of affection or shared activities such as reading or playing games can go a long way towards reducing the child's anxiety and improving his or her well-being. By valuing this emotional role, the caregiver helps parents understand that they are making a valuable contribution to their child's recovery, without having to take on responsibilities that could exhaust them.

Another crucial aspect of managing parents' anxiety is **making them aware of their own well-being**. Emotional and physical exhaustion is a major risk for parents of sick or recovering children. The caregiver must remind them of the importance of taking care of themselves, by offering them respite, however brief. This may involve simple advice, such as resting when they can, asking other family members or friends for help, or taking part in support groups where they can share their experiences with other parents in similar situations. By emphasizing that taking care of themselves is also a way of being there for their child, the caregiver helps them to lighten the emotional burden they are carrying.

It's also helpful to encourage parents to **keep in touch with their outside lives**, be they work, hobbies or other children. Often, a child's illness leads to a total focus on the child, to the detriment of the parents' personal lives. The caregiver can remind them of the importance of maintaining a balance, encouraging them not to neglect their own activities or other family responsibilities. This approach helps to reduce the feeling of overload and preserve a certain normality, essential for their own well-being.

Finally, caregivers need to be alert to signs of **emotional distress** in parents, such as isolation, irritability, discouragement or exhaustion. If these signs appear, it's important to offer extra support, by offering to talk to a psychologist or family counselor, who can help them manage stress and cope with emotional difficulties. The caregiver should always take a proactive approach, anticipating times when parents' anxiety might intensify - for example, before surgery or during a relapse - and offering them reinforced emotional support at these times.

- The importance of creating an environment of trust for the child and his family.

Creating an environment of trust for the child and his or her family is an essential part of caring for young patients, particularly when they are going through a period of illness, rehabilitation or convalescence. Trust is the foundation on which the relationship between the healthcare team, the child and his or her parents rests, and is crucial to ensuring that care takes place in a serene climate conducive to healing and cooperation. When a child feels secure and his or her parents have confidence in the care team, they are more likely to accept treatment, follow medical recommendations, and become actively involved in the recovery process.

The first step in building this trust is to **establish clear, honest communication tailored to each member of the family**. Children, especially the youngest, are often anxious about the unknown, and illness or rehabilitation can seem frightening. As the first line of care, the caregiver must address the child in a reassuring way, using simple words and explaining each step in an understandable way. For example, when it comes to painful or uncomfortable care, it's important not to mislead the child, but to explain what's going to happen, using non-threatening language and insisting that the team will be by his side to make sure everything goes smoothly. This approach helps to reduce the child's anxiety, as he knows what to expect and feels accompanied.

With parents, **transparency** is just as important. Parental anxiety often stems from uncertainty or lack of information. The caregiver must take the time to answer their questions, explain the care provided and the aims of the treatment, and keep them informed of progress, but also of any difficulties. By being honest and available, the caregiver establishes a relationship of trust with parents, who then feel more comfortable asking questions or expressing concerns. This transparency also helps to create a partnership between the care team and the family, involving parents in the decision-making process and reassuring them that their views are taken into account.

Empathy is another essential pillar in creating an environment of trust. Parents, like children, experience moments of great vulnerability when a family member is ill or convalescing. The caregiver must be an attentive and sympathetic listener, acknowledging the emotions of both parent and child without minimizing them. Whether it's fear, sadness, anger or frustration, it's crucial to allow the family to express their emotions freely and receive an empathetic response. For example, if a parent expresses concern about their child's future, the caregiver can take the time to explain the next steps in treatment, while validating the anxiety felt, without trying to minimize it. This acknowledgement of emotions helps to build trust, as parents feel understood and respected.

It's also important to **value the family's involvement** in the care process. Parents know their child better than anyone else, and their involvement in care is invaluable. The caregiver must encourage this participation, whether by asking parents for their views on their child's preferences, involving them in daily care or inviting them to participate in key moments, such as rehabilitation exercises or moments of comfort after care. By actively involving parents, the caregiver shows them that they are an integral part of the care team, and that their role is respected and valued. This also reduces the sense of helplessness often felt by parents in this type of situation, as they have a concrete role to play in their child's well-being.

Creating a **reassuring physical environment** also helps to establish a climate of trust. For children, the hospital or rehabilitation center can be an intimidating place. The caregiver can help make this environment more welcoming, whether by arranging familiar objects in the child's room (such as toys, photos or blankets), or by ensuring that the space is arranged in a way that encourages comfort and safety. The simple act of personalizing the space can make a big difference to the way the child and parents perceive the place of care, making it less foreign and more familiar.

Adapting care to the child's age and abilities is another important dimension of creating this environment of trust. Every child is unique, and his or her needs evolve with age, health and development. The caregiver must be attentive to these specificities and adjust his or her approach accordingly. For example, with a toddler, care needs to be quick and entertaining, while a teenager might prefer a more direct and informed approach. The important thing is always to respect the child's rhythm and preferences, while accompanying him or her with gentleness and patience. This allows the child to feel respected and listened to, reinforcing the relationship of trust with the care team.

Finally, it is essential to **anticipate and prevent moments** of **stress** for the child and his or her family. Through their experience and proximity to patients, caregivers can often identify moments when anxiety is likely to increase, such as before a procedure, during painful care, or when faced with medical uncertainty. By anticipating these moments, they can take steps to alleviate stress, whether through reassuring explanations, distractions for the child (such as a game or a story), or relaxation techniques for the parents. This anticipation helps prevent anxiety from taking over, and maintains a climate of trust and serenity.

Chapter 7

New technologies at the service of rehabilitation

Telerehabilitation: a fast-growing alternative

- How telerehabilitation can support remote patient monitoring.

Telerehabilitation is an innovative approach to supporting remote monitoring of rehabilitation patients, combining technology and personalized care. It has developed as a complementary solution to face-to-face sessions, particularly for patients who find it difficult to travel regularly to rehabilitation centers. Thanks to digital tools, telerehabilitation maintains a constant link between patients and healthcare professionals, while offering greater flexibility in care. It is particularly useful for cardiac, respiratory and neurological rehabilitation, as it enables regular, personalized follow-up at home, while avoiding interruptions in the rehabilitation process.

One of the main advantages of telerehabilitation is that it **ensures continuity of care**, even at a distance. After surgery, an accident or a chronic pathology, rehabilitation often requires regular sessions to maintain or improve functional capabilities. However, for some patients, frequent visits to a rehabilitation center can be difficult, whether for reasons of mobility, distance or personal organization. Telerehabilitation removes these barriers by enabling patients to follow their rehabilitation program from home, while being supervised remotely by healthcare professionals. Thanks to digital tools such as videoconferencing platforms, monitoring applications and connected devices, therapists can supervise exercises in real time, adjust instructions and check on patient progress.

Another major advantage of telerehabilitation is that it offers **great flexibility in the organization of sessions**. Patients can integrate their rehabilitation program into their daily lives more flexibly, choosing the times that suit them best to carry out their exercises. This can encourage greater adherence to the program, as logistical constraints are reduced. What's more, telerehabilitation enables healthcare professionals to personalize monitoring even further, by adapting exercises to the patient's specific needs and rate of progress. For example, a physiotherapist can propose targeted exercises via an online platform, which the patient can follow at his or her own pace, while sending videos or feedback to adjust the sessions according to his or her performance and feelings.

Telerehabilitation also encourages **regular, proactive monitoring** of patient progress. Thanks to real-time monitoring tools, such as motion sensors or applications that collect data on physical performance (heart rate, range of motion, etc.), healthcare professionals can obtain valuable information on patient progress. This data enables them to quickly adjust the rehabilitation program if necessary, taking into account any slowdowns, pain or difficulties encountered by the patient. What's more, this remote monitoring helps to detect signs of aggravation or complications at an early stage, enabling rapid intervention before the situation worsens.

The educational dimension of telerehabilitation is another important asset. This approach is not limited to physical exercise. It also offers an opportunity for therapeutic education for patients, helping them to better understand their pathology, the challenges of rehabilitation and the importance of self-care. Telerehabilitation platforms can integrate educational content, such as explanatory videos, training modules on pain management, or advice on adapting the daily environment to promote recovery. This access to information reinforces the autonomy of the patient, who becomes the actor of his or her own rehabilitation, while remaining accompanied and guided by healthcare professionals.

An essential aspect of **telerehabilitation** is the **reduction of patient isolation**, particularly for those who live far from medical centers or have difficulty travelling regularly. By maintaining a regular link with their therapists and participating in virtual sessions, patients feel less isolated and continue to benefit from guidance and support. This is particularly important for patients with chronic illnesses or the elderly, for whom feelings of isolation can worsen their state of health and reduce their motivation to follow a rehabilitation program. Regular interaction via digital tools helps to maintain a positive dynamic and constant commitment to the rehabilitation process.

Telerehabilitation can also include a **collaborative dimension** between the various healthcare professionals involved in the patient's care. For example, doctors, physiotherapists, occupational therapists and psychologists can more easily exchange information on the patient's progress, thanks to digital information-sharing tools. This collaboration enables better coordination of care, ensuring that the rehabilitation program is comprehensively tailored to the patient's needs, taking into account not only his or her physical progress, but also his or her emotional and psychological state. In this way, telerehabilitation can be part of a multidisciplinary approach, with each professional contributing his or her own expertise to promote a complete and harmonious recovery.

Finally, telerehabilitation offers a **cost-effective solution** for patients, by reducing the costs associated with frequent and sometimes lengthy journeys to rehabilitation centers. It can also relieve overcrowding in healthcare establishments by avoiding unnecessary physical visits, while guaranteeing quality follow-up care. The savings in time and money made by telerehabilitation can also reinforce patient adherence to their rehabilitation program, as they see it as a more accessible approach, adapted to their personal constraints.

- The role of the caregiver in using communication technologies to maintain a link with the patient.

The caregiver's role in using communication technologies to maintain a link with the patient has taken on increasing importance, particularly in the context of modern medicine where digital technologies play a key role in remote monitoring. With the emergence of telemedicine and remote monitoring tools, the caregiver has become a central player in the integration of these technologies to guarantee fluid and continuous communication with the patient, even when the latter is at home. The use of communication technologies not only ensures continuity of care, but also enhances emotional support, encourages patient autonomy, and facilitates the transmission of information to other members of the medical team.

One of the most important aspects of the caregiver's use of technology is the **regular monitoring and follow-up of** patients at a distance. Thanks to videoconferencing platforms, mobile applications and connected devices, the caregiver can maintain regular contact with the patient to check on his or her state of health, ensure that care is being carried out correctly, and respond to any questions or concerns. For example, for a patient undergoing rehabilitation after an operation, regular videoconference sessions enable the caregiver to supervise the performance of exercises at home, give advice in real time, and motivate the patient to continue his or her efforts. This regular link bridges the gap between physical consultations and periods when the patient is alone at home, ensuring the continuity of care essential to recovery.

Remote communication also helps to maintain constant **emotional support**, particularly for isolated or frail patients. Periods of illness, convalescence or rehabilitation can be marked by feelings of loneliness or anxiety, and the regular presence of the caregiver, even at a distance, offers the patient invaluable psychological support. Using communication tools, the caregiver can quickly answer the patient's questions, reassure them about their state of health, and encourage them to persevere in their healing process. For elderly patients or those suffering from chronic illnesses, this close relationship, maintained via technology, helps to reduce isolation and strengthen the human bond despite distance.

Communication technologies also enable caregivers to play a key role **in patient education**. Digital tools facilitate the transmission of educational content, whether in the form of explanatory videos, reading documents or interactive tutorials. The caregiver can, for example, send recommendations for improving the patient's autonomy at home, suggest tips for better pain management, or provide advice on adapting the environment to the patient's needs. This information, shared by the caregiver via technology, helps patients to better understand their condition, manage their day-to-day care, and become more autonomous in the management of their health. The transmission of knowledge is a fundamental aspect of rehabilitation, and technology makes this learning accessible at all times.

Using digital communication tools, caregivers also facilitate the **coordination of care** between different healthcare professionals. In a multidisciplinary approach, where doctors, physiotherapists, psychologists and occupational therapists are all involved in patient care, technologies can centralize information and ensure better coordination. For example, thanks to remote monitoring applications, the caregiver can update data on the patient's condition in real time (such as vital signs, exercise progress or daily observations) and share it with other team members. This enables decisions to be taken more quickly, treatments or exercises to be adjusted in line with the patient's progress, and any gaps in care to be avoided.

Remote monitoring devices, such as motion sensors, heart rate monitors or pain tracking apps, also offer the caregiver valuable tools for monitoring the patient's state of health without requiring a constant physical presence. These tools enable continuous data collection, which the caregiver can then analyze to ensure that the patient is progressing satisfactorily, or to spot early signs of complications. For example, for a patient suffering from heart failure, a connected monitor can alert the caregiver to abnormal variations in heart rate, enabling rapid intervention. These technologies enhance the caregiver's ability to anticipate problems and ensure proactive follow-up, even at a distance.

The use of technology by the caregiver also encourages **active involvement of the patient** in his or her rehabilitation or care. By using interactive applications or online platforms, caregivers can encourage patients to track their progress, record their health data (such as weight, pain, or physical capabilities), and actively participate in their healing process. This fosters patient autonomy, as they become active participants in their own care. The caregiver can then use this information to personalize care and adjust exercises or treatments to the patient's specific needs. This continuous interaction, based on digital communication, strengthens collaboration between the patient and the care team, while increasing the patient's involvement in his or her rehabilitation.

Finally, the caregiver plays an important role **in supporting families** through communication technologies. When patients are cared for at home, their families often play an essential role in providing day-to-day support. The caregiver can use digital tools to maintain a link with the family, informing them of the patient's state of health, giving them advice on how best to support their loved one, and answering their questions. This allows families to feel supported and reassured, while preventing them from feeling helpless in the face of the situation. By using technology proactively, the caregiver ensures better communication with the patient's entourage and fosters a climate of trust, essential to the patient's well-being.

Digital mobility assessment tools

- Use connected applications and tools to assess patient progress (activity bracelets, movement sensors).

The use of connected applications and tools, such as activity bracelets and movement sensors, has revolutionized the way in which patients' progress in rehabilitation or medical follow-up is assessed. These devices enable real-time monitoring and provide objective, precise data on the evolution of patients' physical capacities. By integrating these technologies into the care process, the caregiver can obtain a complete and continuous view of progress, adjust interventions according to the patient's specific needs, and encourage greater autonomy in rehabilitation management. These tools offer a new approach to assessment, combining technology and human support.

One of the major advantages of these connected technologies is their ability to **collect precise data in real time**. Activity bracelets, for example, measure key indicators such as the number of steps taken, distance covered, heart rate and sleep quality. This information, transmitted directly to a dedicated application, enables the caregiver to assess the patient's mobility and analyze his or her level of activity on a daily basis. For patients undergoing rehabilitation after an operation or a chronic illness, this data is invaluable for observing changes in their ability to move around, walk for longer or gradually increase their physical effort. What's more, the ability to track these parameters over a prolonged period provides a global view of progress, enabling care to be adapted as a function of improvement or difficulties encountered.

Motion sensors, meanwhile, are particularly useful in functional rehabilitation. These devices, often integrated into smart clothing or used as portable sensors, accurately record joint and muscle movements. They can detect gesture quality, range of motion and body imbalances. These sensors are particularly useful for assessing patients with motor or neurological disorders, such as those who have suffered a stroke or undergone orthopedic surgery. The caregiver can thus monitor the performance of rehabilitation exercises in real time, correct postures or adjust movements to avoid incorrect compensations, and ensure that gestures performed are in line with physiotherapists' recommendations.

Another important advantage of these tools is that they enable **progress to be visualized and documented**, for both caregiver and patient. Applications associated with activity wristbands or motion sensors offer simple interfaces that display performance in the form of easy-to-interpret graphs or statistics. This enables the caregiver to track improvements over time, identifying periods of stagnation or regression, and adjusting care or exercises accordingly. For the patient, this visualization is also highly motivating: seeing concrete progress, such as an increase in the number of steps taken each day or an improvement in range of movement, boosts self-confidence and encourages continued effort. This visual feedback helps to maintain the patient's commitment to his or her rehabilitation, and gives him or her concrete goals to work towards.

What's more, the data collected by these connected tools enables caregivers **to detect potential complications** or warning signals **at an early stage**. For example, a sudden drop in physical activity, a drop in heart rate or increasingly restricted movements may indicate a problem, such as unreported pain, excessive fatigue or a medical complication. By monitoring these parameters, the caregiver can intervene quickly by adapting the rehabilitation program or alerting the medical team for further investigation. This proactive monitoring is essential to prevent worsening of the patient's condition and ensure safe rehabilitation.

The use of connected applications and tools also makes it possible to **further personalize the rehabilitation program**. Depending on the data collected, the caregiver can adjust the exercises, making them more or less intense, or adapting them to the patient's abilities at a given moment. For example, if the data shows that the patient has managed to walk longer without pain, the walking program can be intensified. Conversely, if the sensors reveal a decline in performance, the exercises can be lightened to avoid physical or mental overload. This personalization of care is a major asset, as it enables us to support patients at their own pace, taking into account their strengths and limitations.

Mobile applications associated with activity bracelets and movement sensors play an important role in **empowering patients**. They enable patients to take an active part in their rehabilitation by tracking their own progress, receiving notifications or encouragement, and setting daily goals. This autonomy strengthens the patient's commitment and enables him or her to better understand the importance of his or her efforts in the healing process. In addition, these applications enable the caregiver to remain permanently connected with the patient, even outside rehabilitation sessions, by receiving alerts in the event of a problem or regular updates on health status. This continuous interaction encourages better adherence to the rehabilitation program.

Finally, connected tools also facilitate **collaboration between different healthcare professionals**. The data collected can be shared with doctors, physiotherapists or other members of the care team, enabling more effective coordination of care. Each professional can consult information on the patient's progress, adjust his or her interventions accordingly, and ensure that the rehabilitation program is coherent and adapted to the patient's overall needs. This multi-disciplinary approach, made possible by connected technologies, guarantees optimal management and improved continuity of care.

  o   Monitor health indicators using computerized, interconnected patient records.

Tracking health indicators using computerized, interconnected patient records represents a major advance in care management, offering more fluid, secure and personalized care for patients. These digital records centralize and update all a patient's medical information in real time, enabling healthcare professionals, including nursing assistants, to monitor health trends accurately, optimize care coordination, and react rapidly when necessary. The digitization of medical records thus enhances the quality of care, while providing a complete and up-to-date overview of the patient's health pathway.

One of the main advantages of computerized patient records (CPR) is their ability to **centralize and organize medical information in a** comprehensive way. Every relevant health indicator, whether vital signs, test results, treatments administered or diagnoses made, is recorded in a single file accessible to all healthcare professionals involved in the patient's care. This centralized system enables caregivers to quickly consult the essential data needed to monitor changes in the patient's condition and adjust care accordingly. For example, by accessing blood test results, blood glucose monitoring for a diabetic patient, or blood pressure data, the caregiver can immediately adapt his or her interventions to the patient's actual needs.

Real-time updating of computerized patient records means greater responsiveness in monitoring health indicators. As soon as a new parameter is recorded, be it a temperature reading, medication dosage or clinical examination, the information is entered directly into the system. This instantaneous update is particularly valuable for patients requiring continuous monitoring, such as those suffering from chronic illnesses or in the post-operative phase. The caregiver can monitor developments in real time and alert the medical team if any indicator falls outside the expected norms, enabling rapid reaction in the event of a deterioration in the patient's state of health, for example by adjusting treatment or requesting an additional examination.

The health indicators tracked via PGDs are many and varied. They include vital vitals (such as heart rate, blood pressure and temperature), laboratory results (blood sugar, cholesterol, etc.), mobility and rehabilitation data for convalescing patients, and information on the patient's mental and emotional state. This information, often recorded in a fragmented way in paper systems or scattered files, is now consolidated in a single digital space. This provides a complete overview, facilitating informed decision-making by the care team. For the caregiver, who is often responsible for the day-to-day monitoring of the patient, this immediate accessibility to key data is a major asset in ensuring continuous, personalized care.

Interconnecting patient records with other healthcare systems **enables optimum coordination of care**. Thanks to this interconnection, data can be shared easily between different departments and healthcare professionals, whether in the same establishment or in different structures. For example, a general practitioner, a specialist, a physiotherapist and a care assistant can all access the same information, facilitating coordinated care and avoiding duplication or errors. This interconnection is particularly beneficial for patients requiring multidisciplinary care. By enabling everyone involved to access the same data, CIOs promote better collaboration between different healthcare professionals, and ensure seamless continuity of care.

Access to computerized patient records also helps **optimize treatment management**. Every prescribed medication, every dose adjustment, every change of treatment is recorded in the file, enabling the caregiver to ensure that therapeutic protocols are followed and to avoid medication errors. If a patient is undergoing a complex treatment, the caregiver can consult the complete treatment plan, check for potential drug interactions, and ensure that medications are administered as recommended. What's more, CIOs facilitate the traceability of care provided, enabling each caregiver to know exactly what care has been administered and when, thereby enhancing patient safety.

One of the major benefits of PGDs is the **prevention of medical errors**. Thanks to the exhaustive recording of a patient's medical history, allergies, current treatments or associated pathologies are clearly visible to all nursing staff. This helps avoid critical errors, such as administering a drug to which the patient is allergic, or repeating unnecessary tests. By accessing this up-to-date information, the caregiver can anticipate the patient's needs and ensure that care is appropriate and safe. For example, before carrying out a treatment, the caregiver can check the IPR for any contraindications, such as allergies to certain dressings or antiseptic products.

CIOs also enable **more accurate assessment of patient progress**. By tracking health indicators on a regular basis and analyzing their evolution over time, the caregiver can measure the patient's progress, identify positive or negative trends, and adjust care accordingly. For example, for a patient undergoing rehabilitation, mobility or range-of-motion indicators can be tracked over several weeks, enabling progressive improvement to be visualized, or periods of stagnation to be identified. These data can then be shared with the rehabilitation team to adjust the exercise program or suggest additional interventions if necessary. This continuous, objective assessment enables care to be tailored to the patient's real needs, while setting realistic, personalized objectives.

Last but not least, the use of IPRs and health indicators **enhances communication with patients and their families**. The information recorded in the file can be explained clearly and in detail, helping the patient to better understand his or her state of health, progress and the actions taken to recover. Caregivers can use this information to provide patients with factual, reassuring information, for example, showing the results of recent tests or explaining changes in vital signs. Moreover, families, who are often anxious about the state of their loved ones' health, can be reassured by the transparency of the information available and by the traceability of the care provided, thus reinforcing their confidence in the care team.

Artificial intelligence and rehabilitation: what place for the caregiver?

- The impact of new technologies on care and rehabilitation methods.

The impact of new technologies on care and rehabilitation methods is considerable, and has profoundly transformed the way healthcare professionals, including caregivers, support patients. These technologies, which include telemedicine, connected devices, artificial intelligence (AI), virtual reality and remote monitoring tools, have opened up new perspectives in patient care. They not only improve the efficiency of care, but also offer more personalized approaches, while enhancing patient autonomy. New technologies provide solutions that make the day-to-day work of caregivers easier, and enable greater responsiveness to the specific needs of each patient, particularly in the field of rehabilitation.

One of the first areas in which new technologies are having a major impact is **telerehabilitation**. Thanks to telecommunication tools, patients can now follow their rehabilitation program at a distance, while remaining in regular contact with healthcare professionals. This is particularly beneficial for patients who live in remote areas or have difficulty travelling. Telerehabilitation enables the caregiver and other professionals to monitor the patient's progress, supervise exercises in real time via videoconferencing platforms, and adjust the program as required. This approach reduces the frequency of face-to-face visits, while ensuring continuity of care. It also avoids interruptions in the rehabilitation process, which is essential for lasting results.

Connected devices such as activity bracelets, motion sensors and heart rate monitors have also become essential tools in rehabilitation. These devices collect real-time data on the patient's state of health, such as the number of steps taken, activity levels, sleep quality and heart rate regularity. This information, recorded in dedicated applications, enables caregivers to monitor the patient's progress continuously and accurately. For example, a caregiver can use this data to ensure that the patient is complying with mobility or exercise instructions, and to adapt care according to observed performance and progress. This remote monitoring makes it possible to detect potential problems, such as a drop in activity or an anomaly in vital signs, and to intervene rapidly if necessary.

New technologies also make it possible **to personalize care** in a much more refined way than ever before. Thanks to artificial intelligence, healthcare professionals can analyze complex data and propose rehabilitation programs or treatments specifically tailored to each patient's individual needs. For example, algorithms can assess a patient's overall state of health, taking into account their medical history, current abilities and rehabilitation goals, and then recommend exercises or treatment adjustments. This approach optimizes the rehabilitation process and improves long-term results. For the caregiver, this translates into more targeted care, a better understanding of the patient's specific needs, and an enhanced ability to respond proactively to his or her evolutions.

Virtual reality (VR) and **augmented reality (AR)** are also redefining the way patients undergo rehabilitation. These immersive technologies offer simulated environments in which patients can perform exercises in a fun and stimulating way. For example, a patient undergoing rehabilitation after a stroke can use virtual reality to practice motor movements in a safe, controlled environment. Virtual reality can make rehabilitation sessions more engaging, overcoming the boredom or frustration that can sometimes accompany repetitive exercises. The caregiver can supervise the use of these technologies, encouraging the patient and helping him or her to make the most of these tools to maximize progress. In addition, virtual reality enables **cognitive rehabilitation**, by stimulating abilities such as attention, memory or coordination, aspects often impaired after trauma or neurological disease.

New technologies have also improved **pain management** during rehabilitation. Transcutaneous electrical stimulation (TENS) or biofeedback devices can be used to control pain and monitor bodily reactions in real time. These tools, often used to complement traditional pain management methods, offer a nondrug alternative to relieve patients, which is particularly beneficial for those wishing to avoid analgesics or who are in the rehabilitation phase after an injury. The caregiver can not only monitor the use of these devices, but also help the patient to integrate them into their daily routine, ensuring that their use is appropriate and effective.

The **digitization of medical records** and the interconnection of healthcare information systems have also had a significant impact on the way care and rehabilitation are delivered. Computerized patient records make it possible to track health indicators in real time, archive all test results, and facilitate communication between the various professionals involved in patient care. This interconnection is particularly useful for rehabilitation patients, who often require multidisciplinary care involving doctors, physiotherapists, psychologists and care assistants. Thanks to these digital systems, all members of the care team can access the same information, exchange recommendations, and coordinate care more fluidly and efficiently. This improves continuity of care, and enables the rehabilitation program to be adjusted rapidly according to the patient's progress.

New technologies also encourage **greater involvement of patients in their own rehabilitation**, making them active players in their own health. Thanks to mobile applications and monitoring platforms, patients can track their progress, record their results, and access advice in real time. This empowerment motivates patients to be more involved in their rehabilitation and to take initiatives to improve their health. By guiding them in the use of these tools, the caregiver plays a key role in encouraging this proactive approach and ensuring that the patient makes correct use of the technologies made available to them.

Finally, **patient education** has also benefited from new technologies. Interactive platforms, explanatory videos and online training modules enable patients to learn more about their condition, their treatment and the exercises to follow. This educational dimension, accessible at any time, reinforces patients' understanding of their rehabilitation process and enables them to adopt more responsible and informed behaviors.

- The importance of keeping up to date with technological advances to optimize patient care.

In an ever-changing medical world, it is essential for healthcare professionals, including nursing assistants, to remain trained and informed about technological advances in order to optimize patient care. Technological innovation is rapidly transforming care practices, bringing with it new methods, tools and approaches that can significantly improve the quality of care, patient safety and treatment efficacy. Keeping up to date with these developments not only enables us to respond better to patients' needs, but also to offer more personalized, faster and more comprehensive care. The role of the caregiver, often on the front line of daily patient care, is evolving in parallel with technological advances. It is therefore crucial to master these new technologies in order to make the most of them and guarantee care that is adapted to the demands of modern medicine.

One of the main benefits of ongoing training in new technologies is to enable caregivers **to make effective use of the digital and connected tools** that are increasingly being integrated into healthcare. Whether it's computerized patient records, connected devices such as activity bracelets or motion sensors, or remote monitoring applications, these technologies require a technical understanding to be fully exploited. With proper training in these tools, the caregiver can not only monitor the evolution of the patient's state of health more accurately, but also make better use of the data collected to adjust care in real time. This means greater responsiveness to the patient's needs, particularly for detecting abnormalities or adapting the pace of rehabilitation. For example, a caregiver capable of analyzing the data provided by a movement sensor can quickly adjust rehabilitation exercises according to the patient's actual performance, thus optimizing each session.

Regular training courses also enable new skills to be acquired in relation to innovations such as **virtual reality (VR)**, **augmented reality (AR)** or **assistive robots**. These technologies, which are beginning to revolutionize rehabilitation and patient support, require in-depth knowledge of how they work if they are to be effectively integrated into care. For example, the use of virtual reality for motor or cognitive rehabilitation requires familiarity with specific software and devices in order to adapt them to patients' needs. A caregiver trained in these new methods will be able to supervise virtual re-education sessions, reassure patients about their use, and provide additional support by maximizing patient engagement and motivation in these immersive environments. Similarly, mastery of assistive robots, designed to help mobilize patients or provide care assistance, will enable caregivers to offer safer support, while lightening certain physical tasks.

Keeping abreast of technological advances also helps to **improve communication and care coordination**. With the widespread use of computerized and interconnected patient records, medical information management has become a central element of patient care. Being able to use these systems with ease enables caregivers to better integrate the care they provide within a multidisciplinary team. Every piece of data recorded in these files, whether test results, vital signs or clinical observations, must be correctly interpreted and shared with all healthcare professionals. Appropriate training ensures that the nursing auxiliary masters these information management tools, thus guaranteeing optimal traceability of care and fluid communication between the various players involved in patient follow-up. What's more, this helps to avoid errors, improve continuity of care, and guarantee more consistent and secure care.

Ongoing training in new technologies also helps to strengthen the **relationship of trust with patients**. In a context where patients are increasingly exposed to new medical technologies, they may express concerns or questions about their use. A trained and informed caregiver is better able to answer patients' questions, reassure them about the efficacy and safety of these devices, and encourage them to use them optimally. For example, a rehabilitation patient who uses a connected device to monitor his or her progress may feel anxious about the technology if he or she doesn't fully understand it. A trained caregiver can clearly explain how the device works, how it helps improve rehabilitation, and how the patient can track his or her own progress to stay motivated. This reassuring interaction reinforces the patient's commitment to their care.

In addition, regular training courses **keep** caregivers **up to date on the safety and ethical protocols** associated with the use of new technologies. With the rise of connected devices and the massive collection of healthcare data, the issue of confidentiality and protection of patients' personal information has become paramount. Caregivers, as professionals handling this sensitive information, need to be aware of the security standards and regulations in force. Keeping abreast of developments in this field helps to ensure that patient data is handled responsibly, respecting confidentiality rules and minimizing the risk of leakage or misuse of information.

Finally, continuing education is essential to **prepare for the future** of **healthcare**, which is rapidly evolving under the influence of technological innovations. Personalized medicine, treatments based on artificial intelligence, and new remote monitoring devices are just a few examples of the advances already transforming the sector. By staying up to date and anticipating developments, caregivers are better prepared to adopt these technologies as soon as they are introduced into routine practice. This enables them not only to remain competitive in the job market, but above all to offer cutting-edge care that meets the needs of an increasingly connected and informed population.

Conclusion

A vocation in the service of rehabilitation

- Summary of the challenges and rewards of the trade.

The nursing profession is both demanding and deeply rewarding, combining daily challenges with human rewards. It's an essential profession in the healthcare system, where the caregiver is often on the front line, accompanying, caring for and supporting patients at what can be a very difficult time in their lives. While the complexity of this profession can sometimes seem overwhelming, the rewards often come from the direct and tangible impact the caregiver has on the well-being of patients, and the personal satisfaction that comes from this unique relationship with those who need it most.

One of the **main challenges** of the nursing profession is the **physical and emotional demands** of daily work. Patient care can be physically demanding, involving tasks such as mobilizing bedridden patients, helping with toileting, or providing support when moving around. Working staggered hours, including nights, weekends and public holidays, adds another dimension of difficulty, with fatigue that can build up over time. On an emotional level, the caregiver is often confronted with situations of great vulnerability: patients at the end of life, intense physical suffering, or families in distress. In such situations, the caregiver has to manage his or her own emotions while offering empathic support to others, which can be particularly challenging.

Another challenge is the **workload**. In many facilities, care assistants have to deal with large numbers of patients, often understaffed, which can make it difficult to give individual attention to each patient. They have to juggle a number of tasks while respecting deadlines and medical protocols. The pressure can be intense, especially in fast-paced hospital environments where emergencies can arise at any moment. Maintaining impeccable quality of care in these conditions calls for rigor, resilience and effective stress management.

Despite these challenges, the nursing profession offers priceless **rewards**. One of the greatest satisfactions is to see the direct impact of one's actions on patients' quality of life. The simple act of providing a little comfort, alleviating pain, or enabling a patient to regain a degree of autonomy brings immense gratification. These gestures, sometimes seemingly modest, can transform a patient's daily life. For example, helping a patient to walk again, to eat on their own, or to perform simple acts of daily living, reinforces the caregiver's sense of usefulness and pride in accompanying a person towards better health or greater dignity.

Human relations are another of the profession's major rewards. By being in direct contact with patients, orderlies forge bonds of trust and affection with them. This proximity enables them to establish a dialogue, sometimes without words, which helps them to understand the patient's needs beyond simple clinical observation. These human relationships bring richness and meaning to daily life, especially when patients, or their families, express gratitude for the care they have received. This positive emotional feedback is often a great source of motivation for caregivers.

The nursing auxiliary profession also enables them to **develop genuine expertise**. Through experience, caregivers acquire the technical and relational skills that make them indispensable in the care chain. They learn to quickly detect signs of deterioration in a patient's state of health, to adapt care to specific needs, and to work closely with nurses, doctors and other members of the medical team. This expertise, recognized by colleagues and patients alike, reinforces a sense of professional pride.

What's more, the caregiver profession offers a **diversity of practices**. Caregivers can work in a variety of environments, from hospitals to retirement homes, home care or rehabilitation centers. This diversity enables them to vary their approach to care, to accompany patients in very different situations, and to continually adapt their skills to the needs of each workplace.

Another rewarding aspect of the job is the **psychological support** caregivers provide to patients. Through their presence, attentiveness and benevolence, orderlies play a key role in providing emotional support to sick or frail people. They are there not only to provide physical care, but also to reassure, allay fears and bring comfort at what are often difficult times. For many patients, the relationship with the caregiver becomes an important anchor, and the caregiver can feel a deep sense of satisfaction in knowing that he or she is helping to soften these moments of vulnerability.

- Encouragement and a call to commit to this rewarding path.

Choosing to become a nursing auxiliary means choosing a deeply human path, where every day is an opportunity to provide precious support to those who need it most. It's a career that, while demanding, is also immensely rewarding on a personal level. Working as a caregiver is more than just a job: it's a vocation, a commitment to others, a dedication to improving the lives of vulnerable, sick or frail people. It's a profession where even the simplest daily gestures can make a huge difference to the well-being and dignity of patients.

One of the finest aspects of this profession is the **richness of human relations**. As an orderly, you are at the heart of care, in direct contact with patients. You develop a relationship of trust, support and sometimes even friendship. You're the one who's there to listen, to comfort, to support in moments of doubt or suffering. The special bond you create with your patients is a source of deep satisfaction. A patient's smile, a sincere thank-you, or simply the knowledge that you've brought a little comfort in a difficult time - these are priceless rewards that give meaning to your work.

This **profession** is also a **source of continuous learning**. Every patient is different, and every situation teaches you something new. You develop technical skills, but also human ones, such as patience, listening, empathy and emotional management. You learn to adapt your care to each situation, to recognize the subtle signs of a positive evolution or deterioration in a patient's state of health, and to collaborate with other healthcare professionals to offer the best possible care. This wealth of experience allows you to grow, not only as a professional, but also as an individual.

Choosing to be a caregiver also means accepting **daily challenges**. The work is sometimes difficult, physically and emotionally demanding, but it is precisely in these challenges that the beauty of the profession lies. The moments of fatigue or stress are counterbalanced by the small victories: seeing a patient gradually regain his or her autonomy, helping an elderly person feel dignified despite illness, supporting a loved one in the darkest moments. Those moments when you know that your actions, your gestures, your presence have had a real impact on someone's life are sources of immense pride.

What's more, this profession offers you the **chance to contribute to positive change** in society. In a world where the demand for care continues to grow, particularly as the population ages, caregivers are needed more than ever. By committing yourself to this path, you join a community of professionals dedicated to providing quality care, respecting human dignity, and improving the daily lives of the most vulnerable. Your work is essential, not only for patients and their families, but also for the smooth running of the entire healthcare system. It's a commitment that, every day, helps to make the world a little more humane and a little more supportive.

For those hesitating to embark on this career, it's important to understand that the caregiver is not just a technical carer, but also an **emotional pillar** for many people. You are the one who accompanies patients in moments of vulnerability, helps them overcome their fears and pain, and provides comfort when they need it most. This closeness and humanity are at the heart of this profession, and they will bring you immense emotional richness.

Finally, it's important to remember that the nursing profession offers a wide range of **career prospects**. If you choose this path, you'll never be locked into a single role. With time, experience and further training, you'll be able to rise to positions of responsibility, move into other healthcare professions such as nursing, or specialize in specific areas such as geriatrics, rehabilitation or palliative care. The possibilities are vast, and this career can be the starting point for a long and rewarding journey within the medical field.

Appendices : Practical resources and tools

- Practical sheets: protocols, mobilization techniques, evaluation grids.

1. Hand hygiene

- **Objective**: Prevent nosocomial infections.
- **Equipment**: Hydro-alcoholic solution or antiseptic soap.
- **Technology**:
    1. Wet hands with water (if soap).
    2. Apply a dose of soap or hydroalcoholic solution.
    3. Rub palms, backs of hands, between fingers, under fingernails and around thumbs.
    4. Rinse with clean water (if soap).
    5. Dry with a clean towel (if soap and water).
    6. Use a towel to turn off the tap.

2. Taking vital signs

- **Objective**: Assess the patient's clinical condition.
- **Constants to be measured** :
    1. **Body temperature**: Use a thermometer (ear, forehead, mouth or rectal, depending on the situation).
    2. **Heart rate (pulse)**: Palpate at wrist (radial), neck (carotid) or foot (pedal). Count pulses for 60 seconds.
    3. **Respiratory frequency**: Observe breathing (inspiration/expiration) and count cycles for 60 seconds.
    4. **Blood pressure**: Use a blood pressure monitor (automatic or manual with stethoscope). Record systolic/diastolic pressure.

Practical guide: Mobilization techniques

1. Mobilization of a bed-ridden patient (without standing)

- **Objective**: Prevent bedsores and maintain joint mobility.
- **Equipment**: Slip sheets or lift if necessary.
- **Technology**:
    1. **Side roll**: Turn the patient onto his or her side, keeping hips and shoulders aligned. Use a sheet to facilitate movement.
    2. **Moving into a sitting position**: gently lift the patient into a sitting position on the edge of the bed, while supporting the back and shoulders.
    3. **Mobilization of upper and lower limbs**: Perform gentle flexion and extension movements at joints (ankles, knees, elbows, wrists).

2. Mobilization with standing

- **Objective**: To help the patient stand upright, improve circulation and muscle tone.
- **Equipment**: Transfer belt, walker or lift.
- **Technology**:
    1. Position the patient on the edge of the bed, with feet on the floor.
    2. Place the transfer belt around the patient's waist.
    3. Keeping the back straight, help the patient to stand up by supporting him/her with the belt and using the walker if necessary.
    4. Ensure balance and encourage small, safe movements.

Practical info: Evaluation grids

1. Pain assessment grid (VAS - Visual Analog Scale)

- **Objective**: Evaluate the intensity of pain felt by the patient.
- **Tool**: Ruler or visual cursor from 0 (no pain) to 10 (maximum pain).
- **How to use** :
    1. Ask the patient to rate his or her pain on the scale.
    2. Interpretation :
        - 0 to 3: Mild pain.
        - 4 to 6: Moderate pain.
        - 7 to 10: Intense to unbearable pain.

2. Autonomy evaluation grid (ADL - Activities of Daily Living)

- **Objective**: Measure the patient's degree of autonomy in essential activities.
- **Elements evaluated** :
    1. **Mobility**: getting up, walking, lying down.
    2. **Toilet**: Ability to wash oneself.
    3. **Feeding**: Ability to feed oneself.
    4. **Dressing**: Ability to dress oneself.
    5. **Incontinence**: Managing urinary and fecal functions.
- **Notations** :
    1. 0: Independent.
    2. 1: Partial assistance.
    3. 2: Total assistance.

3. Norton scale (pressure sore risk assessment)

- **Objective**: Identify patients at risk of pressure sores.
- **Criteria assessed** :
    1. **General condition**: Good, fair, poor.

2. **Mobility**: Mobile, immobile, very immobile.
3. **Awareness**: Alert, apathetic, unconscious.
4. **Incontinence**: None, occasional, frequent.
5. **Diet**: Good appetite, eat little.
- **Interpretation** :
    1. Score ≤ 14: High risk of pressure sores.
    2. Score > 14: Low risk.

Practical guide: Pressure sore prevention techniques

1. Regular position change

- **Objective**: Reduce prolonged pressure on support points.
- **Frequency**: Every 2 hours.
- **Technology**:
    1. Alternate positions (dorsal, left lateral, right lateral).
    2. Use cushions to relieve pressure areas (heels, sacrum, elbows).

2. Use of anti-bedsore mattresses or cushions

- **Objective**: distribute pressure evenly and reduce the risk of pressure sores.
- **Equipment**: Dynamic air mattresses, gel cushions or viscoelastic mattresses.
- **How to use** :
    1. Place the patient on the mattress/cushion.
    2. Regularly check the integrity of the skin in high-risk areas.

These practical examples can serve as a quick reference for caregivers and the medical team, to ensure safe, comfortable and effective care. They facilitate the application of protocols, while ensuring rigorous, personalized patient follow-up.